Communication Skills for Doctors

Communication Skills for Doctors:

A guide to effective communication with patients and families

By

Peter Maguire

Honorary Consultant Psychiatrist and Director, Christie CRC Psychological Medicine Group, Manchester, UK

ARNOLD

A member of the Hodder Headline Group
LONDON
Co-published in the USA by
Oxford University Press, Inc., New York

W 64

COMMUNICATION
PATIENT - MEDICAL
STAFF RELATIONS
INTERPERS REL

First published in Great Britain in 2000 by
Arnold, a member of the Hodder Headline Group
338 Euston Road, London NW1 3BH

http://www.arnoldpublishers.com

Co-published in the United States of America by
Oxford University Press Inc.,
198 Madison Avenue, New York, NY10016
Oxford is a registered trademark of Oxford University Press

British Library Cataloguing in Publication Data
A catalogue record for this book is available from the British Library

Library of Congress Cataloging-in-Publication Data
A catalog record for this book is available from the Library of Congress

ISBN 0 340 66309 X

1 2 3 4 5 6 7 8 9 10

Commissioning Editor: Fiona Goodgame
Development Editor: Sarah de Souza
Production Editor: Anke Ueberberg
Production Controller: Fiona Byrne

Typeset in 10pt Sabon by Phoenix Photosetting, Chatham, Kent
Printed and bound in Great Britain by Redwood Books Ltd, Trowbridge

CONTENTS

PREFACE

It was assumed that as a medical student and then as a junior doctor I would acquire communication skills by watching my consultants at work. I was also taught that if I genuinely appeared to care for patients, both they and their relatives would disclose their key problems, whether they be physical, social, psychological or spiritual in nature.

I soon learned that these assumptions were incorrect, since the consultants on whom I was modelling myself had not received any formal training in communication skills. For example, when breaking bad news they used routinized and logical approaches. I vividly recall spending two hours with a man who insisted that his wife should not be told her cancer had advanced and she did not have long to live. Despite all my efforts to highlight the reasons why he should change his mind about this, he remained adamant. I realized then that meeting strong emotion with logic was no solution.

Later, as a Casualty Officer, I often had to deal with very angry patients or relatives, sometimes just after the relative had been bereaved. I felt most ill equipped for these tasks, and often failed to diffuse the anger and emotional pain.

Thus it became clear that being 'caring, nice and logical' is not enough when dealing with the difficult communication tasks that are commonly encountered by senior medical students and junior doctors at the sharp end of clinical practice. Even the essential task of assessing patients' problems can be practically and emotionally taxing unless the senior student or doctor knows how to make optimal use of the time they have available, identify key problems and the associated feelings accurately, and help to resolve these difficulties.

Recently, more attention has been paid in medical training to helping students and doctors to acquire key communication skills. Even so, my experience of assisting with such training has revealed that many senior medical students and junior doctors still feel ill equipped to deal with important communication tasks such as breaking bad news, assessing suicidal risk and having a dialogue with a confused patient.

The guidelines contained in this book are designed to help senior medical students and doctors to become much more confident and effective in handling these key communication tasks.

Peter Maguire

INTRODUCTION

This book is aimed at senior medical students and young doctors in training. The key objective is to help them to become more competent in dealing with common communication tasks which they find particularly difficult. The book is also designed to help them to develop a more proactive style of interviewing than the current non-directive methods that are emphasized.

Chapters 1, 2, 3 and 4 are concerned with examining basic aspects of common obstacles to effective communication between doctors, patients and relatives. Guidelines are then suggested on how they may adopt a much more efficient method of interviewing which nevertheless leaves patients feeling understood and satisfied. Separate advice is included for the provision of information, as it has been found that acquisition of information during interviewing requires quite separate skills to those needed to help patients to recall accurately and understand the information they have been given.

In Chapter 5, attention is also given to issues that arise in relation to interviewing key relatives. This includes handling some of the more difficult situations in which relatives are demanding and there is family conflict.

The rest of the book deals with more complex situations about which medical students and senior doctors say they receive too little help during their training, although they encounter such scenarios frequently. The topics covered include breaking bad news, handling patients who are distressed, distinguishing between normal and abnormal reactions, and handling anger and hopelessness.

Chapter 8 is devoted to communicating with withdrawn patients, discussing the common reasons for withdrawn behaviour and the management of the different situations that may arise. Chapters 9 and 10 deal with more emotionally charged issues concerning assessment of suicidal risk and helping relatives who have been bereaved. In the latter chapter particular attention is given to what young doctors experience when they have to break sudden and unexpected bad news either in hospital or in the home.

If doctors are to interview effectively and therefore to get close to the reality of the suffering of patients and their families, they need to know how to be able both to do this and to survive emotionally. The final chapter is therefore devoted to discussion of doctors' personal survival.

The topics that have been chosen for inclusion are those that senior medical students and young doctors repeatedly tell us in workshops they need most help with, but about which they receive little guidance during their training.

chapter 1

IMPROVING YOUR INTERVIEWING

INTRODUCTION

During your medical training you will have been taught how to take a history and interview patients. You should also have been given guidance on how to handle other communication tasks. However, it is unlikely that you will have been given sufficient guidance about strategies to help you handle more difficult communication situations such as breaking bad news, dealing with angry patients and relatives, attempting to obtain a history from withdrawn patients, assessing patients at risk of suicide, and communicating with the relatives of patients who have died suddenly and unexpectedly either in hospital or at home.

There is therefore a risk that you will seek to keep your interviews emotionally neutral by ignoring cues about patients' worries and emotions. Importantly, this can lead patients to avoid mentioning key problems. These and other barriers to effective communication are discussed in Chapter 3.

Traditionally, doctors are taught to use a directive style of interviewing. This involves them asking patients what their main complaints are and then asking rote questions about the presence or absence of specific symptoms (e.g. 'Have you had any problems with your breathing?' or 'Any problems with your waterworks?'). Unfortunately, this approach has been found to be relatively ineffective in promoting patient disclosure, and key problems may not be revealed. An interviewing style that seeks to elicit signs and symptoms of physical illness but also demonstrates a genuine interest in the patient as a person early in the interview, and seeks to cover physical and psychological aspects, is much more effective in promoting honest disclosure (Stewart *et al.*, 1995). This interviewing style is reviewed in Chapter 4.

Before considering how to handle the important communication tasks described in this book, you need to be aware of some general principles about interviewing and doctor–patient communication. These include the following.

- Importance of the interview
- Managing time
- Establishing trust
- Delaying fixing things

contd

- Building a partnership
- Making educated guesses
- Allowing for culture
- Picking up cues
- Checking

IMPORTANCE OF THE INTERVIEW

The medical interview is crucial for identifying the exact problems for which patients need help. The history contributes far more to accurate diagnosis than do medical investigations. Moreover, it is the task that you will perform most frequently during your medical career. It is therefore crucial that you feel competent at interviewing the patient.

How you elicit a history has a profound influence on patients' level of disclosure and their subsequent compliance with your offered advice and treatment. It can also have a strong effect on patients' expectations of subsequent encounters with health professionals. For example, if you restrict your enquiry to physical aspects, then you will educate patients to the effect that you are a 'physically orientated' doctor and are not concerned with other aspects of their predicament. They may then withhold any social or psychological problems, and they will tend to believe that other members of your team, such as nursing staff, are also only interested in the physical aspects of illness.

Similarly, if psychiatrists focus solely on eliciting psychological problems, patients will be less likely to mention any key physical illnesses or symptoms.

MANAGING TIME

Most doctors work under formidable time constraints. Therefore you need to interview in a way that ensures you make maximum use of the time available, but also leave patients and relatives feeling that they have been listened to and their main problems have been identified and understood. There is a risk that the patients you see first in a clinic, on a hospital ward or on a home visit will be given more time than those you see later. You should therefore learn to ration your time and distribute it equitably. This can only be done if you are prepared to decide how much time you have available for a given task, and negotiate this with the patient as described in Chapter 5. The negotiation of realistic time limits educates patients that you do not have unlimited time available. This encourages them to make maximum use of your time and to disclose key problems earlier. In contrast, if you do not give patients any indication of the time available, they may believe that they have plenty of time and react badly when you seek to terminate the interview. When you have negotiated the time available it is much easier to close your interviews on time and explain what you would like to do next.

Health professionals often fear that if they mention the limited amount of time available, patients will be angry or irritated and less likely to co-operate. In practice, the opposite is the case. Setting time limits will alert you to patients who might be more demanding than is reasonable. Thus if you explain to patients that they have one hour for an interview, and they immediately complain that this is not long enough, this may indicate that they are needy and potentially emotionally dependent. Most patients, on hearing that they have an hour for the interview, worry that they do not have enough of interest to say to fill the time.

When you educate patients about the time available you should adhere to this time limit. You therefore need to be prepared to interrupt patients before the end of the interview and warn them that the interview is coming to a close, recap what you have learned, and check whether the patient has anything to add. Otherwise, important information may be left undisclosed. If patients offer you new information at the end of an interview, it is important to acknowledge this but not to be seduced into extending the interview. Instead, you should arrange to meet them as soon as possible to clarify the new information.

ESTABLISHING TRUST

A commonly held view is that you must give patients time to 'thaw out' before they can be expected to disclose their main problems. Doctors who hold this view spend time conversing socially with patients before they attempt to take a formal history. While time spent in social conversation may feel comfortable, it educates patients that the doctor is delaying eliciting their main problems. Patients come for help with a need to talk about their problems, rather than to spend time in irrelevant conversation. Focusing immediately on their problems helps patients to feel more secure and also clearer about what they are meant to talk about. You are more likely to foster trust by saying 'Can you tell me just why you have come to see me today?' than by asking whether they saw last night's television programmes.

DELAYING FIXING THINGS

When doctors enter medicine they usually do so because of a genuine wish to cure patients of their illnesses and problems. This motivation to fix patients' problems as soon as possible can create difficulties. The moment a doctor hears a patient disclose a problem he or she may seek to resolve it without checking whether there are any other important problems that the patient has not yet disclosed (Beckman and Frankel, 1984). This can lead to major problems going unrecognized and untreated at both the initial and subsequent consultations. It is important to say, for example: 'So, you have been getting this pain in your calves on walking and becoming breathless. Before I discuss these further, are there any other problems you would like to mention?' If the patient has a lengthy problem list, you can ask them to put their problems in order of priority and explain that you will deal with the most important one first, rather than seek to try to deal with all of them. Patients will usually be understanding about this.

BUILDING A PARTNERSHIP

There is a temptation that doctors may believe they are the 'strong professionals' caring for dependent patients, and therefore they are responsible for making all key decisions. Yet regarding your relationships with patients as partnerships, and seeking to educate them that this is the case, has major benefits in terms of disclosure of their problems by patients and subsequent compliance. From the outset you need to demonstrate your willingness to negotiate with patients. Thus you should ask routinely 'Is it all right if I take notes to help me remember what we discuss?' or 'Can I start by taking you back to the time when your problem first began? Is that OK?' Such negotiation may lead patients to say they are not prepared to go through a lengthy history 'for the tenth time'. Instead, they want to talk about their immediate problems. You should respect this.

During an interview, patients may become distressed when describing upsetting events such as a bereavement or worries about their illness. Instead of insisting that they continue to talk about that event or worry, you should check whether they are able and willing to say any more about it ('I can see this is distressing for you – can you bear to say any more about it just now?'). This gives the patient permission to indicate that the event or worry is too painful to talk about, and it helps you to avoid pushing them too far and causing them intolerable emotional pain. They will therefore feel more secure in their relationship with you, and they may later feel strong enough to talk about the event or worries in more detail.

When you acknowledge patients' distress overtly you also educate them that you are alert to their feelings.

MAKING EDUCATED GUESSES

As you talk with patients you can gain strong intuitions about how they are feeling despite their verbal statements. For example, a patient may claim that she is coping well with her multiple sclerosis, but you get a strong hunch that she is deeply distressed about the resulting disabilities. It is of no help to her if you keep this intuition private. Instead, trust your intuition and mention it directly: 'You say you are coping well with your illness, but as we talk I get the feeling you are very distressed about the way it is preventing you from living a normal life.' The patient may respond by confirming how disabled she is and how distressing this is for her. Alternatively, she may explain that your guess is incorrect and say more about the actual impact of the illness on her life. It does not matter if your guess is incorrect. It educates patients that you are trying to further your understanding of their predicament. This is a major step in developing trust and showing empathy with your patients.

ALLOWING FOR CULTURE

You will, of course, meet patients from diverse backgrounds and cultures. It is particularly important to negotiate with people from different cultures as to whether the procedures you plan to follow in your interview are acceptable to them or not. For example, it may be that the family will not allow you to be alone with the patient, in which case you should accept this.

When trying to assess the impact of particular illnesses and treatments, it is useful to check whether coming from a particular culture has affected the way in which the patient has responded to the illness or treatment. Some illnesses and treatments are experienced as much more stigmatizing by patients and relatives from different cultures.

PICKING UP CUES

However well you try to interview, you should remember that it is a percentage business and you will never get it completely right. You may, for example, be tired and miss certain cues that a patient gives. Most patients will repeat their cues if the topic is important, and give you a further chance to acknowledge and explore them. The key is to write down verbal and non-verbal cues as the interview progresses, so that you can check through your notes and see whether you have explored them with the patient before the interview ends. When patients feel that their cues have been acknowledged, they will speed up their disclosure rate, and this will make the interview more efficient and effective.

CHECKING

If at any stage in the interview you feel that you have not understood what the patient has said, it is important to explain this and to invite them to clarify the information (e.g. 'I got the impression your father died three years ago, but I now realize I am wrong about that. Could you tell me exactly when he died?'). Patients will accept such clarification because they realize that you are trying your best to gain a proper understanding of their experiences.

SUMMARY

If you are willing to follow these general principles, you will find that interviewing becomes an enjoyable and worthwhile exercise. Patients will give you positive feedback about how helpful they have found you and how much they feel you have understood their problems.

REFERENCES

Beckman, H.B. and Frankel, R.M.C. 1984: The effect of physician behaviour on the collection of data. *Annals of Internal Medicine* 101, 692–6.

Stewart, M.A., Belle Brown, J., Wayne Weston, W., McWhinney, I., McWilliam, C. and Freeman, T. 1995: *Patient-centred medicine: transforming the clinical method.* Thousand Oaks, CA: Sage.

chapter 2

PSYCHOLOGICAL BARRIERS TO COMMUNICATION

INTRODUCTION

A major objective of the medical interview is to ensure that patients disclose all of their main problems, whether these are physical, social or psychological in nature. Otherwise, they are more likely to feel dissatisfied with the care given and less likely to comply with the advice and treatment offered (Stewart, 1995). If major concerns remain undisclosed, patients will cope less well with their illness and treatment, and will be at greater risk of developing high levels of emotional distress and even clinical anxiety and/or depression (Parle *et al.*, 1996).

Unfortunately, patients often fail to disclose all of their main problems. In particular, they tend not to disclose the true impact of their illness and treatment on their daily functioning, mood and personal relationships. Yet the development of major depression or anxiety impedes recovery from physical illness in general and surgery in particular and has been associated with a higher mortality rate.

OBJECTIVES

This chapter will consider:

- why patients do not disclose key problems;
- the tactics doctors use to keep the consultation in 'safe waters';
- the reasons they do so.

Before you read the chapter you should pause and reflect on what you consider might be the possible reasons for patients not being honest with the doctor about their problems, and how doctors might themselves contribute to non-disclosure.

REASONS FOR NON-DISCLOSURE

PATIENTS' CONTRIBUTION TO NON-DISCLOSURE

Patients' reasons for non-disclosure:

- Problems are inevitable and cannot be alleviated
- Chances of survival might be reduced
- Fear of being labelled neurotic
- Desire to protect the doctor
- Not legitimate to mention non-physical problems
- Negative response to cues
- Selectivity of disclosure

Problems are inevitable and cannot be alleviated

Patients with chronic disabling diseases (e.g. rheumatoid arthritis) or life-threatening diseases (e.g. cancer or heart disease) believe, albeit wrongly, that any adverse physical side-effects of treatment or psychological difficulties such as body image problems and high levels of distress are an inevitable consequence of their predicament. They believe that these problems must be the price they have to pay for treatment of their disease, and so they feel that there is no point in mentioning them as they cannot be alleviated.

Chances of survival might be reduced

When a patient is told that the treatment they are receiving is necessary to save their life, they may be frightened to mention any adverse effects because this might result in the treatment being reduced in dosage or stopped altogether. When the doctor asks them if they are experiencing any side-effects, they then minimize or even lie about them. For example, a woman who was being treated with adjuvant chemotherapy for breast cancer developed severe nausea and exhaustion. When she was asked about any side-effects she said she was having very little trouble. However, for most of the month after treatment she was too exhausted to get out of bed and she was too sick to eat much. When asked why she had not disclosed this to the clinician, she said she was terrified that her chemotherapy would be stopped and that her disease would recur and she would die.

Fear of being labelled neurotic

Patients who become very distressed and feel that they are struggling to cope with their illness and treatment may be especially loath to admit this to their doctor. They fear that they will be labelled as 'pathetic, inadequate and neurotic'. They also worry that they will be perceived as ungrateful for the care they have been given, and that these judgements will result in their receiving second-class care.

Desire to protect the doctor

The nature of the relationship between the patient and doctor can affect disclosure profoundly. When patients have come to like their doctor, they also become concerned about the doctor's welfare. They are then more likely to try to protect him or her from the reality of their predicament by avoiding disclosing problems that could be very distressing. For example, a 25-year-old woman had a colostomy performed because of severe ulcerative colitis. She was very grateful to the surgeon concerned because of the substantial symptom relief she experienced. However, she developed profound body image problems which severely affected her day-to-day functioning. She became reluctant to go out of the house, and would not risk developing close relationships because she feared rejection. However, she did not feel able to tell the surgeon about these problems because she thought he would be distressed that his surgery had had such an effect on her.

Patients are also often sensitive to doctors being under considerable work pressures and appearing hassled. This may also lead them to withhold key problems.

Not legitimate to mention non-physical problems

Patients say that a major reason for non-disclosure is that they do not believe it is legitimate to mention problems other than those strictly related to their illness and treatment. They claim that doctors do not ask them explicitly about their own perceptions of their illness, the prognosis, and related concerns and feelings. Instead, they usually ask 'What have you been told already?' Yet there may be little relationship between what previous doctors have said to the patient and the patient's awareness of what is wrong and what their prognosis may be. Patients also report that doctors do not usually ask them about how they have reacted psychologically to the diagnosis and key treatments, and what the impact has been on their mood, daily lives and personal relationships.

For example, when patients have undergone major surgery, such as the removal of a breast, they say it is rare for them to be asked by anyone involved in their care how they felt about the surgery and how they have reacted to it. In the absence of such explicit enquiry, they believe that doctors are not interested in learning about the effect of the surgery on them. Therefore they feel that it is not legitimate to mention any problems spontaneously.

Negative response to cues

Despite the lack of active enquiry by doctors about non-physical aspects of their predicament, a substantial minority of patients still provide verbal or non-verbal cues. Thus they may mention at some point in the consultation that they are 'upset' or 'worried' about their illness, treatment or prognosis. They may also appear quite upset. Unfortunately, they may find that doctors are reluctant to acknowledge their cues and to explore them any further. This reinforces their feeling that it is not legitimate to mention these other aspects.

Selectivity of disclosure

Since patients feel that when they are discussing their problems with the physician or surgeon they are only entitled to disclose physical problems, they will not disclose other concerns spontaneously. Psychiatrists can experience the opposite problem. Because they may focus on questions about a patient's psychological adjustment, the patient may start to believe that they are not interested in any concomitant physical illness.

DOCTORS' CONTRIBUTION TO NON-DISCLOSURE

Studies of consultations between doctors and patients have confirmed that patients' claims about the areas on which doctors prefer to concentrate are correct. First, they do not usually ask questions which seek to elicit patients' perceptions of their predicament (e.g. 'What do you make of what is going on?') or their reactions to the diagnosis and treatment (e.g. 'How has all this affected you in yourself?'). Moreover, these studies have found that when patients do provide explicit cues about social and psychological problems, the doctors use strategies designed to limit or block further disclosure, known as *distancing strategies* (Maguire *et al.*, 1996). Common distancing strategies are listed below.

Distancing strategies used by doctors:

- Selective attention to cues
- Normalizing
- Premature reassurance
- False reassurance
- Switching the topic
- Passing the buck
- Jollying along
- Physical avoidance

Selective attention to cues

When the patient volunteers a number of problems which relate to physical, social and psychological problems, the doctor focuses solely on the cues about physical problems. In the following example, a surgeon is reviewing the progress of a woman who underwent a mastectomy for breast cancer 3 months previously.

MR F: How have you been getting on since I saw you last?

MRS P: OK, I think. I am able to move my arm all right and comb my hair. I am not having any more pain, but I have been worrying about . . .

MR F: I am pleased that your arm is much better and that you have no pain now.

Not only did the surgeon fail to pick up the patient's cue that she was worried, but he interrupted before she could explain what she was worried about. Had he asked her she would have revealed that she was terrified that her cancer would recur because two of her close friends had had bad experiences. One had already experienced an early recurrence, and the other had died. This selective attention to cues about physical problems is common. Some patients try to cope with it by repeating their cue – 'I have been worried' – several times before they give up.

Normalizing

In the course of their work, doctors see many patients and relatives who are distressed. It is therefore easy to become habituated to this and to believe that it is a normal consequence of physical illness and treatment. There is then a danger that patients' distress is dismissed as normal, and this can block disclosure. For example, a 26-year-old woman was admitted to hospital with a threatened miscarriage. She and her husband had been trying to have a baby for 8 years. On entering hospital she was very upset and emotional. The admitting doctor responded by saying 'Of course you are upset, you are bound to be. I am sure you will soon settle down'. His response made her feel that he was not interested in her worries. She was terrified that her husband would leave her if she did not deliver a healthy baby. However, in the face of the doctor's use of normalization she did not feel able to reveal this concern, and remained very distressed. When she subsequently miscarried she coped badly.

Premature reassurance

People become doctors because they wish to help to relieve patients' suffering. They generally therefore seek to offer practical help as soon as possible within a consultation. The danger of this is that they will try to 'fix' a problem before they have checked whether the patient has any other problems. Such premature reassurance can prevent disclosure of other major problems. For example, a 25-year-old woman presented to her general practitioner with complaints of pain in her lower back which was radiating down her left leg. The doctor immediately asked questions to clarify the exact nature of her back problem, and he then examined her. The examination confirmed that she had a disc problem. He then gave her appropriate advice before ending the consultation. In reality she had had the back problem for some months, and her reason for presenting was her concern that she had started to bleed between periods and she was extremely worried about this, as she was afraid she had cervical cancer. However, she was frightened to mention this at the outset of the consultation, lest her fears be proved correct. Cancer was not diagnosed until 6 months later.

False reassurance

A major objective of any consultation is to try to leave patients with hope even when their predicament is serious. However, this can lead to doctors protecting patients from facing reality by offering false reassurance. In the following example a young man re-presented to a neurologist because he was worried that his multiple sclerosis had recurred and that he was suffering a serious deterioration in his physical health and ability to function.

DR B: I gather from your doctor's letter that things haven't been good lately.

MR S: They haven't. I am finding it increasingly difficult to get my left leg to work. I am getting pins and needles in my left arm and I am having to use a stick to try and walk. I am scared I am going to be bedridden before much longer.

DR B: Oh come on, I think you are being far too pessimistic. We are not at that stage yet.

The inability of the neurologist to confront this patient with the probable reality of further deterioration prevented the patient from disclosing his fears. These fears were based on what he had learned about what had happened to other patients with multiple sclerosis while he was in hospital during his original admission.

Switching the topic

When doctors are talking to patients who raise a potentially distressing topic, there is a danger that they will switch the focus of the conversation to a safer, more neutral subject. In the following example, a 50-year-old man presented to a cardiologist complaining of chest pain and breathlessness. There was a strong history of heart disease in his family.

DR B: How bad has your breathlessness been?

MR M: I can only walk 50 yards before I have to rest. I can't get my breath and my chest pain gets too much.

DR B: What's this pain in your chest like?

MR M: It's a gripping pain, as if my chest is being squeezed in a vice. I am terrified I am going to die. Am I going to die?

DR B: Apart from the breathlessness and chest pain you mentioned, have you experienced any other problems?

The cardiologist was not aware that he had switched the topic. However, his switching prevented the patient from divulging why he was so terrified of dying. All of the male relatives in his family had died between the ages of 50 and 52 years from heart attacks, and he was convinced that the same thing was going to happen to him.

A common form of switching is to move the focus away from the patient on to the family. In the following example, a general practitioner was talking to a patient with diabetes about the fact that her blood sugar levels were out of control, and emphasizing that she must comply with the advice offered to her.

DR W: So, things have been pretty erratic with respect to your blood sugar control recently?

MRS J: Yes. I am terrified I am going to suffer, go blind or have a stroke.

DR W: How have your family been managing?

The general practitioner spent a further 5 minutes talking to the patient about her family, and never returned to her fear of these complications and why she was worried about them.

Passing the buck

When a doctor cannot answer the patient's question because of a lack of knowledge, or perceives that this is not his or her area of expertise, it is appropriate to suggest that the patient consults a more senior colleague. However, the doctor may well have the answer but be reluctant to respond honestly. Instead, he or she will pass the buck, for example by saying 'I think you should ask the consultant'. This strategy ignores the fact that patients are trusting the doctors with difficult questions because they believe they will receive a helpful answer, and it leads the patients to feel even more worried and frustrated.

Jollying along

To help the patient to adjust better, their doctor may try to cheer them up if they notice that they are looking miserable or worried, by saying 'Come on, there is no need to look so glum'. For example, when a young doctor was walking through a ward he noticed a man who had been admitted with a relapse of multiple sclerosis and was looking miserable. He already knew from talking to him that he was a keen football fan and supported Manchester United. In a genuine bid to cheer up the patient he said 'Come on, cheer up, you know the game is on tonight – it should be a cracker'. Although the patient knew that Manchester United were playing in an important European cup game in the evening, he remained preoccupied with fears that he was not going to return to independent living because he had become incontinent of urine and had noticed a marked drop in his sex drive.

A better way of tackling the same situation would have been for the doctor to walk over to the patient and say 'Look, I can see you are worried. Would you like me to come back and talk to you later? I have to go and see one or two other patients just now'. The patient is likely to have said yes. The doctor could then have returned and asked the patient why he was so worried. The patient would have disclosed his concerns, and the doctor could have reassured him that it was unlikely that these disabilities were permanent, and that they were probably just part of a temporary relapse.

Physical avoidance

Doctors know that they should try to talk with their patients, but they may find themselves avoiding this situation because it may be too distressing (e.g. talking to a young girl who is dying from a brain tumour). They may try to explain this away on the grounds that they are too busy, as in the following example.

A 21-year-old woman was admitted to hospital 2 days after her twenty-first birthday complaining of severe headaches. She complained that light was very painful and she had been vomiting. Investigations confirmed that she had meningitis, and despite urgent antibiotic treatment she did not respond. She went into a coma and was transferred to intensive care, where her parents maintained a vigil by her bedside. The registrar responsible for her care knew he ought to talk to the relatives about her situation. However, he felt that he could not face doing this because he was distressed and did not know what to say. His avoidance intensified the relatives' uncertainty about what was happening, and led them to think that there might have been some negligence on the part of the hospital. When the patient died, the parents complained that they had received insufficient support and explanation about what was happening.

These distancing strategies are commonly used, yet doctors wish to care for their patients and help them to recover from disease and minimize suffering. Therefore there must be good reasons why they use these distancing strategies (Parle *et al.*, 1997).

DOCTORS' REASONS FOR DISTANCING

Reasons for distancing

- Fear of harming patients psychologically
- Fear of being asked difficult questions
- Fear of getting too emotionally close
- Doubts about the value of medicine
- Fear of taking too much time
- Concern about personal survival
- Lack of training in communication skills
- Lack of support
- Lack of validation

Fear of harming patients psychologically

Doctors fear that if they ask direct questions about patients' views of their illness and their reactions to their illness and treatment, this could unleash strong emotions such as anger or despair which they will not be able to contain. They worry that this will harm the patient, cause greater distress, and lead some patients to give up altogether and even die prematurely. For example, a doctor may feel that asking a young woman with AIDS how she sees her illness working out will lead her to become very distressed and to talk about her fear that she will die within the next year or so. Although the doctor fears that this will be counter-productive, the young woman will in fact feel grateful that someone is showing an interest in her view of her predicament and giving her an opportunity to voice her concerns and feelings. The therapeutic value of helping patients to voice their concerns and associated feelings, even when their concerns cannot be resolved, is discussed in the next chapter and in Chapter 7.

Fear of being asked difficult questions

Doctors fear that if they try to explore their patients' concerns about their predicament, those patients may ask them difficult questions such as 'Am I dying?', 'How long have I got?' or 'Why didn't you diagnose it sooner?' Such questions are difficult to handle even if the doctor knows the most appropriate strategies to use. Doctors also fear that admitting they do not have an answer will create more problems and make them feel that they have failed through not being able to give a clear response to the question.

Fear of getting too emotionally close

Finding out how the lives of patients and their families have been affected by chronic disabling, degenerative or life-threatening diseases brings doctors close to their patients' real suffering. This will inevitably be distressing. If doctors are constantly confronting such painful situations, they may worry that this is threatening their own emotional survival, unless they know how to deal with these situations constructively and to cope with the stress involved (see Chapter 11).

Doubts about the value of medicine

Doctors are trained to believe that they should be able to identify and resolve their patients' problems, and that their job is to make things better. It is therefore difficult for them to face patients when they cannot cure the illness or alleviate suffering. This may lead them to question the value of medicine in general and their own role in particular.

Fear of taking too much time

Doctors commonly believe that if they enquire about patients' concerns, especially those related to psychological and social aspects, this will take up too much time and hinder their ability to identify and deal with the patients' physical problems. They also often believe that if they focus on the patient's agenda rather than taking a standard medical history, this will take far too much time. In reality, starting with the patient's main problems allows doctors to use their time much more effectively, and it will be much more likely that they will identify their patient's main problems and achieve better patient satisfaction, compliance and recovery.

Concern about personal survival

For all of these reasons doctors worry that their own personal survival will be jeopardized if they try to communicate in depth, rather than focusing solely on physical aspects of disease, ignoring the social and psychological aspects and using distancing tactics to keep the conversation in 'safe waters'.

Lack of training in communication skills

Many doctors recognize that they have received insufficient training in how to interview effectively and manage the difficult communication tasks that they commonly encounter, such as having to break bad news and deal with the resultant distress and strong emotions like anger or despair.

Lack of support

It has been found that even if doctors have acquired the relevant interviewing skills, and have confidence that their use will benefit patients and relatives, they may still be reluctant to use them if they feel unsupported by their colleagues. Thus doctors need to feel that they will receive practical assistance if, as a result of their more effective interviewing, they uncover more complex problems than they feel they can cope with. They also need to feel that they are cared for as individuals by their supervising colleagues, otherwise they will continue to use distancing strategies.

It can be difficult to adopt this more holistic approach when senior colleagues give negative feedback. In the following example, a surgeon has asked the house officer to give feedback about how a woman is feeling 4 days after her mastectomy.

MR B: It is now what, 4 days since she had her mastectomy. How is she getting on?

DR J: Her wound has been draining well. She is doing OK physically, but she feels devastated at losing a breast and is very low in her mood.

MR B: Yes, of course, many women are upset initially, but let's concentrate on her physical recovery. We haven't time for all that other stuff.

Dr J felt confused by this response. He had learned during his training that it was important to check the emotional impact of major surgery, yet Mr B had dismissed this. He had to forge a good relationship with Mr B in order to foster his own career.

Lack of validation

Few doctors and medical students have experienced positive feedback about the value of exploring all of their patients' problems even when they can do little to resolve them. They therefore tend to assume that if a patient is distressed at the end of a consultation, that consultation must have gone badly.

In the following example, a senior medical student clerked a newly referred out-patient who had presented with symptoms suggestive of angina. The student found that the patient's father had died of a sudden heart attack when she was 7 years of age. At this point the patient became upset and started to sob. She disclosed that she had felt deserted by her father and had never grieved since that time. The student was concerned that the patient was so upset, and said 'I am sorry if I have upset you'. However, the patient responded positively, saying 'In a funny way I feel a great burden has been lifted. It is the first time I have ever talked about it. I have always worried I would drop dead like he did. That's why these pains have worried me so much'.

SUMMARY

Patients often fail to disclose major problems to the doctors who are caring for them. Both patients and doctors contribute to this. Patients are looking for active signals that it is legitimate to disclose their concerns, whilst doctors are utilizing distancing strategies to keep the consultation in 'safe waters'.

The next chapter will discuss strategies that can help doctors to relinquish these distancing strategies and improve their ability to elicit their patients' concerns.

REFERENCES

Maguire, P., Faulkner, A., Booth, K., Elliott, C. and Hillier, V. 1996: Helping cancer patients disclose their concerns. *European Journal of Cancer* **32A**, 78–81.

Parle, M., Jones, B. and Maguire, P. 1996: Maladaptive coping and affective disorders in cancer patients. *Psychological Medicine* **26**, 735–44.

Parle, M., Maguire, P. and Heaven, C. 1997: The development of a training model to improve health professionals' skills, self-efficacy and outcome expectancies when communicating with cancer patients. *Social Science and Medicine* **44**, 231–40.

Stewart, M.A. 1995: Effective physician–patient communication and health outcomes: a review. *Canadian Medical Association Journal* **152**, 1423–33.

chapter 3

ELICITING PATIENTS' PROBLEMS

INTRODUCTION

To overcome the barriers to patient disclosure discussed in Chapter 2 it is necessary to follow three principles. These include patient-centred rather than doctor-centred interviewing, integrating physical with other modes of enquiry, and using a proactive rather than a non-directive interviewing style.

> **OBJECTIVES**
>
> The objectives of this chapter are:
>
> - to discuss principles of interviewing;
> - to describe the key skills to be used;
> - to highlight the areas to be covered.

When you follow these principles and utilize the strategies suggested it is much more likely that patients' key problems will be elicited, their perceptions of their problems and reactions established, and the impact on their daily lives, mood and personal relationships clarified. This will enable you to make more efficient use of your time and improve patient satisfaction and compliance.

GUIDING PRINCIPLES

PATIENT-CENTRED INTERVIEWING

As was mentioned in Chapter 2, doctors have traditionally been taught to use a directive style which involves asking patients what their main complaints are and then following these up with questions about the presence or absence of relevant key symptoms. The main aim is to identify the nature of the physical or mental illness from which they are suffering. However, this traditional approach is relatively ineffective in promoting disclosure. An interviewing style which both focuses on eliciting symptoms and signs of illness and shows genuine interest in patients as individuals, their reasons for seeking help, their perceptions of what might be wrong, their feelings about this and the impact of any problems on their daily lives, mood and personal relationships is more effective, leading to greater patient compliance with advice and treatment, as well as to greater patient satisfaction (Stewart, 1995).

INTEGRATING MODES OF ENQUIRY

As discussed in Chapter 2 doctors' emphasis on physical or psychological aspects at the outset of the consultation may programme the patient to believe that the doctor is only interested in the physical or psychological aspects of their predicament. In contrast, showing an interest from the outset in both physical and psychological aspects of the patient's situation will educate them as an individual that you are interested in the impact of illness and treatment on their personal life, as well as the nature of their illness. Thus a surgeon may, when taking a history of a breast lump, not only ask how it was found but what the woman thought it was and how she felt about it. This immediately educates the woman that the surgeon is interested in her perceptions and reactions.

PROACTIVE INTERVIEWING STYLE

The barriers to disclosure described in Chapter 2 will only be overcome if you use certain interviewing skills which will be discussed in the next section. If you simply ask the patient what their problems are and listen for a few minutes without making any response, they will not know for sure that you have been listening. They may then fear that you are already making negative judgements about what they are saying, and the rate of disclosure will be correspondingly low (Bensing and Sluijs, 1985).

It is commonly feared that if doctors interrupt patients while they are giving a general account of their symptoms, this will be perceived as intrusive and interrogatory. In reality, the lack of an active response by the doctor conveys to the patient that the doctor is not really interested in what they are saying. If the doctor then tries to follow this 'initial paragraph' approach with more detailed questions, the patient may have already decided that the doctor is not really interested, and so will not respond.

APPROACHING THE INTERVIEW – CHOICE OF STRATEGIES

SCENE-SETTING

When you have sufficient time you should seek to take a full history of the patient's problems, establish how key problems began, how these have developed subsequently, what investigations and treatments have been carried out and the patient's views of and reactions to these. This will enable you to gain a good understanding of how and why the patient is currently adjusting to their predicament, and the problems that need to be addressed.

PROBLEM-SOLVING

When you have between 5 and 15 minutes to assess a problem, or if the medical condition is overriding, it is important to focus on the patient's current problems and to check which is the major one, so that it is covered in the limited time available.

HOW TO BEGIN THE INTERVIEW

If patients are being seen in a consulting room, it is important that you stand up as each patient enters, establish eye contact, move towards them and greet them verbally with a clear 'Hello' or 'Good morning', using the patient's correct name and title. You should then indicate by words and gestures where the patient should sit. The chairs should be placed facing each other, rather than behind a desk. You should then sit down and adopt a posture that conveys interest and friendliness while avoiding extremes such as lounging back in a casual manner or moving so close to the patient that he or she feels intruded upon. You should then introduce yourself by name and explain your status. When patients are in bed it is important to greet them in the same way and then to sit in a chair close to the bedside so that you are at the same level as the patient. You should ensure that you are not interrupted by leaving your bleeper with other members of staff.

ORIENTATING THE PATIENT

What is going to be covered

Begin by explaining what you intend to cover (e.g. 'I would like to find out as much as possible about your present problems in the time we have available'). Mentioning problems in the plural encourages the patient to realize that they can talk about several problems rather than just one.

Explaining the time limits

Indicate how much time you have available, as this helps patients to make an effort to ensure that they have disclosed their main problems in the available time. You should always have an idea of the amount of time you have available when assessing patients, given your knowledge of your overall workload. This will make it less likely that patients will leave disclosing important problems until the end of the interview, and it reduces the risk that patients will become dependent on you because they feel that they have unlimited time. Even so, it is important that you check with the patient that he or she is content with the amount of time mentioned. Some patients will complain that the time offered is too short. In that case, you can explain that although everything may not be completed on this occasion, they can meet with you again soon to complete the interview. In most cases this results in the patient focusing on the problems that they need to disclose. Moreover, there is evidence that they feel that doctors and students who have mentioned the time limits are more empathic towards and interested in them (Thompson and Anderson, 1982).

Explaining note-taking

You should explain that you wish to take notes to help you remember what was discussed, and you must add that these will be confidential. Most patients are reassured by seeing you write down the key information that they are disclosing instead of just nodding. If a patient indicates that they do not want certain information recorded, it is important to explore their reasons. It is also important to check whether they are still prepared to talk.

DR K: Can I ask you about your current problems?

MR L: (looking distressed) I am not happy about this.

DR K: Why are you unhappy?

MR L: I thought I was going to see the consultant.

DR K: As I explained, I am his registrar. He asked me to talk to you to get a history so he can then concentrate on working out what needs to be done next. We will be seeing him together later. Is that all right?

MR L: I suppose so.

DR K: Are you prepared then to tell me what has been happening to you?

MR L: Yes.

OBTAINING A FULL HISTORY

The following areas should be covered to obtain a full history.

- The nature of key problems
- Clarification of these problems
- Date and time of onset
- Development over time
- Precipitating factors
- Help given to date
- Impact of the problems
- Availability of support
- Patients' views of their problems
- Attitude to similar problems
- Screening questions

THE NATURE OF KEY PROBLEMS

The doctor's first task is to help patients to communicate the nature of their current problems. Each problem should be properly clarified before you move on to any other topic. You should always allow for the possibility that initial disclosure is masking the problems that the patient is most concerned about. Once you have elicited the patient's main problems, you should summarize them by saying, for example, 'So far, as I understand it, you have been increasingly breathless, have felt very tired and have been coughing up blood. You have been worrying that this might mean you have lung cancer. Before I go into these symptoms in detail, have there been any other problems that you have not yet mentioned?' In doing this you should be aware that the patient may have problems in physical, social, psychological or spiritual domains. This use of a screening question ('Is there anything else you have not yet mentioned?') minimizes the likelihood that important problems will remain disclosed.

It is important to check which problem the patient would like to start with ('Which of these would you like to tell me about first?'). In most instances, patients start with the problem which is perceived by the doctor to be the most important on medical grounds. If it is evident that one of the problems mentioned is potentially life-threatening you should negotiate with the patient to start with that one, rather than the problem which the patient volunteers.

CLARIFICATION OF THESE PROBLEMS

You should actively clarify the exact nature, intensity and duration of each problem ('What exactly is your pain like? How bad is it? How long does it last?').

DATE AND TIME OF ONSET

You should take care to date exactly when each of the main problems started. Patients can date events accurately provided that they are encouraged to do so, and you must not accept too easily that patients find it difficult to remember. The use of anchor dates such as birthdays, anniversaries or other events can help them to do this ('Was this close to any key events in your life, like a birthday or anniversary?').

DEVELOPMENT OVER TIME

You should next find out how each problem has developed over the period between onset and the current interview. You should be especially alert to any major changes in the intensity and frequency of a problem, as such 'change points' may provide important clues to the aetiology of these difficulties.

PRECIPITATING FACTORS

It is important to check whether the patient has any views about causation of the onset of illness and any change points. Patients tend to search for meaning even when no causal event has occurred. This can result in their falsely relating the onset of current problems to unrelated events. Thus a 54-year-old former business executive gave a history of frequency of micturition, thirst and tiredness. He insisted that it began after he was made redundant. A careful history ('When did your problem with passing water begin?') established that he had developed these symptoms over a year before his redundancy ('When exactly were you made redundant?'). His tiredness and impaired work performance had led him to be selected for redundancy.

False attribution may also occur when the event which triggered the illness was upsetting and the patient prefers to avoid thinking about it. They may then implicate a more neutral event. For example, a 25-year-old man attributed a severe asthma attack to a recent bout of flu. However, a relative informed the doctor that he had developed asthma within a few weeks of his mother's death. Therefore you should date the onset of key problems and possible precipitants independently, and cross-check the dates if you still have doubts.

HELP GIVEN TO DATE

Many patients are already on treatment or have undergone previous treatment. It is therefore important to try to establish the exact nature, dose and duration of each treatment given, and to check whether the patient has noticed any change in relation to each treatment. It is particularly important to ask about any adverse side-effects and to establish their nature and severity, otherwise patients will minimize these ('Have you experienced any problems since you started treatment – any problems at all?').

IMPACT OF THE PROBLEMS

You must ask directly if the patient's problems have been having adverse effects on their ability to work, to cope with day-to-day chores, and to pursue their hobbies, leisure and social activities.

You should also ask about the impact of the problems and any treatments on the patient's mood and personal relationships ('How has your angina affected your mood? How has it affected your relationship with your wife?').

AVAILABILITY OF SUPPORT

The amount of practical and emotional support that patients perceive they are receiving influences how they cope psychologically. Patients' perceptions of how much practical and emotional support they have received in relation to their current problems should be established ('How do you feel about the support you have been getting?'). They should also be asked if they have confided in anyone about their problems ('Have you spoken to anyone about this?').

Families' reactions can vary from being too understanding and protective to being completely disinterested and intolerant.

PATIENTS' VIEWS OF THEIR PROBLEMS

Patients should be asked what they think is wrong with them ('What do you make of your pain and tiredness? What do you think it might be due to?'). They should also be asked how they consider things will work out ('How do you see things working out?'). Unless you are aware of how the patient perceives the situation and how they envisage their problems working out, you will not be able to pitch reassurance at an appropriate level.

ATTITUDE TO SIMILAR PROBLEMS

In order to put the patient's problems and attitudes into perspective, you need to find out whether they have experienced similar problems before. If they have done so, you should clarify for each episode whether there was any particular trigger, how the problem affected them, how long it lasted and what, if any, treatments they responded to. This will allow you to decide whether the patient is vulnerable to particular types of physical or mental problems, and whether they are susceptible to particular stresses. For example, in a patient with recurrent depression it may become evident that each episode was triggered by a loss event such as bereavement. This information will also enable you to determine whether the episodes are clinically different, and to predict what treatments will be effective.

It is important to check how well the patient was functioning before the onset of their present problems, otherwise you may set unrealistic goals for treatment and fail to realize that prior impairment of functioning was due to other factors.

For example, a 55-year-old man presented with a history of severe rheumatoid arthritis. He claimed that it was causing him to become house-bound and making his life miserable. However, the doctor established that even before the onset of his rheumatoid arthritis this patient had not been going out of the house, due to his becoming depressed after the sudden and unexpected death of his wife, and the subsequent development of a severe depressive illness.

SCREENING QUESTIONS

However well you try to establish patients' current problems they may actively withhold them as discussed in Chapter 2. It is therefore important to summarize the problems that have been disclosed, and then to check whether there are any other problems that have not yet been mentioned.

KEY SKILLS TO BE USED

It has been established that the use of specific interviewing behaviours promotes patients' disclosure of their problems (Goldberg *et al.*, 1993; Maguire *et al.*, 1996).

Skills that promote disclosure

- Acknowledging and exploring verbal cues
- Non-verbal cues
- Open directive questions
- Open to closed cones of questions
- Establishing and maintaining eye contact
- Being empathic
- Making educated guesses

contd

- Summarizing
- Negotiation
- Control
- Precision

ACKNOWLEDGING AND EXPLORING VERBAL CUES

As you begin to ask patients about their presenting complaints, they will give important verbal cues about the nature of these complaints and their impact on their life. It is most important that you respond immediately by acknowledging and exploring these cues further. This educates the patient that you are really interested in what they are saying.

Dr S: So, what has brought you to see me today?

Mrs C: I have been having terrible problems with my knee again. It has become swollen and very painful. I am finding it very difficult to put any weight on it. It is increasingly hard for me to walk any distance. I am scared it is not going to get any better.

Dr S: So, you are worried about your knee being swollen and very painful, and hindering your ability to walk, and frightened it won't get any better.

Mrs C: Yes.

Dr S: Can I explore your knee problem in more detail?

Mrs C: Yes.

Dr S: What concerns you most about your knee at the moment?

Mrs C: The pain, it's getting intolerable.

Dr S: Can you tell me more about the pain it's causing. What exactly is the pain like?

By moving in and immediately asking about these cues, the doctor signals a real interest in what the patient is going through. Had he just allowed her to continue talking for a few minutes before interrupting, she would have believed he was only interested in obtaining a superficial account of her experiences.

NON-VERBAL CUES

Patients often give hints of other problems by changes in their tone of voice, facial expression, posture or expression of feelings. You should be alert to these and acknowledge them ('You seem angry' or 'You look upset – can you bear to say why?').

OPEN DIRECTIVE QUESTIONS

In giving an account of key complaints, patients may not spontaneously disclose their perceptions of what is going on and their resultant feelings. They may also not be open about their reactions and feelings concerning key treatment events and outcomes. You should therefore use open directive questions to educate the patient that you are interested in their feelings and perceptions. For example, a patient may be asked 'When you first coughed up blood what did you think was going on?' or 'When you learned you had rheumatoid arthritis, how did you feel?' or 'How has treatment been going?' They are then likely to give important cues about their perceptions and feelings, and these should be acknowledged and clarified as advised earlier ('You say you were shocked at having a colostomy. Can you say more about this?'). This educates the patient that you genuinely want to understand their predicament and what they are going through.

OPEN TO CLOSED CONES OF QUESTIONS

Here the patient has given the doctor a broad indication of the nature of the probable problem. The doctor then asks questions related to his or her professional agenda to elicit whether or not the problem is of the kind he or she thinks it is.

DR D: You say you have been having severe pain in your abdomen. Can you tell me exactly what it has been like?

MRS S: It is a terrible gripping pain. When it comes on it is like a hand crushing me inside. It has been getting unbearable.

DR D: How frequently are you getting these pains?

MRS S: They are coming more often. It is now every 20 or 30 minutes.

DR D: Does the pain go anywhere else?

MRS S: No.

DR D: Have you had any problems with sickness?

MRS S: No.

DR D: Have you had any problems with your bowel habits?

MRS S: I have not been to the toilet for 3 days now.

In this case, questions are being asked to elicit whether there is a particular physical problem with the patient's bowels. The patient accepts these questions as relevant because they relate to her major complaint, and they reassure her that the doctor or student is familiar with what she has been experiencing.

ESTABLISHING AND MAINTAINING EYE CONTACT

If patients are to disclose their problems, they need to feel that they are being listened to and understood. The establishment of eye contact with the patient at the outset of the interview, and maintaining it at reasonable intervals throughout the consultation, is most important. Patients do not expect you to look at them all the time, particularly when you are writing notes. However, if at any stage they say something particularly important, they expect you to re-establish eye contact with them. Otherwise, they will not believe that you are interested in what they are saying. It can be difficult to take notes and maintain eye contact, but the secret is to look up at the patient during any important utterances.

BEING EMPATHIC

Patients are much more likely to disclose their key problems and associated feelings if they feel that you have some understanding of their situation. You can best indicate this by being genuinely empathic and sharing your feelings about the patient's predicament ('No wonder you are so bitter that you had a heart attack when you made all this effort to keep yourself fit and took your diet very seriously').

MAKING EDUCATED GUESSES

Many doctors and students have important intuitions about how patients are feeling, and they often realize that what the patient is disclosing does not match their own impressions of the problem. However, they are frequently loath to share this concern in case their guess is wrong and the patient becomes angry. You should therefore be prepared to share your educated guesses, as patients are usually grateful when you try to further your understanding of the situation. If the guess is wrong, they will be prepared to correct you. The educated guess should be put in a tentative way so that the patient can refute or correct it if necessary.

DR P: As we are talking I get the feeling that you are not coping anything like as well as you are claiming since you learned you had diabetes.

MRS M: Yes, you are right, I am very upset. I am terrified I am going to go blind like my grandfather.

SUMMARIZING

Patients need to feel that they have been listened to. Summarizing and reflecting back their complaints educates them that you are listening. It also gives them the chance to correct you if you misunderstood what they have been saying.

DR M: As I understand it you have been feeling very anxious. You have been worrying that you have a brain tumour because of headaches you have been getting, and you have been feeling confused.

MR P: It is not just confusion. I have been hearing voices saying there is a plot to kill me and that my mother is an impostor.

NEGOTIATION

In Chapter 2 it was stated that doctors fear that patients may become too distressed if they talk about certain aspects of their illness and treatment. There is no way in which you can tell whether or not it is safe to ask a patient about particular aspects of their problems. Instead, you should negotiate with them if you feel it is likely that they are going to find some problems too painful to discuss. This negotiation should be genuine and should indicate to the patient that they can say no if they feel it will be too distressing to talk about specific topics.

DR P: You tell me you have been having a lot more attacks of asthma since your father died.

MISS A: I had virtually no attacks in the year before he died, but in the last 6 months they have been getting more frequent.

DR P: Can you bear to tell me how he came to die?

If the patient indicates that she is not willing to do so, Dr P should accept this and then check what she would like to talk about next.

CONTROL

It is usually easy to get most patients talking about their problems, but it can be more difficult to keep them from wandering off the point and wasting time. Your level of control is optimal when the patient has been given enough time to respond to key questions but does not take too long or wander off the point. Patients will only focus in this way if they are encouraged to do so.

It is important that you explain to the patient at the beginning of the interview that your main task is to elicit their current problems. If they start to talk about irrelevant matters they can be reminded of this ('What you say is interesting, but is it relevant to my understanding of your current problems?').

You may worry that such interruptions are unacceptable to patients, as they might well be in social conversations. However, patients usually welcome this redirection because it signals that you wish to know about their current problems. Patients with obsessional personalities may insist that they are allowed to tell their story in a lengthy and pedantic way. Even in these cases, you should attempt to keep them to the point and work within the available time slot, as such patients can often be speeded up and encouraged to give an accurate story within reasonable time limits.

PRECISION

Patients often tend to give data that is vague, especially when they are ill and suffering. You should therefore explain that it is important for them to be precise about the information they are providing, as it will help you to determine more accurately what is wrong and what help is needed. Any inconsistencies or uncertainties in the information that they supply should be checked immediately. Thus you might say 'I am still confused about when your problems started. Can we get this clear?' It is also helpful to ask for exact examples of the problems the patient has volunteered. 'You say you have been suffering from blackouts. Can you describe exactly what happens when you experience one of these?'

AVOIDING INHIBITORY BEHAVIOURS

Behaviours that inhibit disclosure

- Premature advice
- Premature reassurance
- Closed questions
- Leading questions
- Narrow focus

In addition to the use of premature advice and reassurance described in Chapter 2, there are other behaviours that inhibit patient disclosure (Goldberg *et al.*, 1982; Maguire *et al.*, 1996).

CLOSED QUESTIONS

Questions which merely invite a yes or no answer inhibit disclosure, yet they are commonly taught as essential to history-taking. Thus questions such as 'Any problems with your waterworks?' or 'Any problems with sleep?' will generally invite a one-word answer, and the patient will not usually elaborate further.

LEADING QUESTIONS

A leading question is one which invites a specific answer. For example, when a surgeon says to a patient after surgery, 'Everything is going well, isn't it?', it is difficult for the patient to admit that things are far from well and there have been major complications.

NARROW FOCUS

If the early part of the history focuses on physical aspects alone, the patient will be persuaded into believing that the doctor is only interested in physical aspects. Similarly, if the doctor only shows an interest in psychological aspects, the patient will believe that he or she is not interested in their physical problems.

ONCE THE PROBLEMS HAVE BEEN ESTABLISHED

RECAPITULATION

Once you have elicited the patient's problems and examined the patient physically (and, where appropriate, examined the mental state), you should summarize their main problems.

DR D: Can I check with you that I have got things right? Your main problem has been your stomach pain, and you fear you might have bowel cancer like your father. You have had no response to the drugs given to you for irritable bowel, and this has made you worry even more that it must be cancer.

MRS S: Yes.

SCREENING QUESTIONS

Despite the use of all of these techniques, it is possible that the patient may still have withheld important concerns. You should therefore ask a screening question to check this ('Before I explain what I think might be wrong with you, what you told me and what I have found on examination, can I just check if there is anything you would like to add to what you have told me? Are you sure?').

EXPOSITION AND TERMINATION

Often you will not be in the position of having clear information to give the patient after obtaining an initial history. You will therefore need to be honest with the patient about this and the need for further tests.

DR D: OK we have got a few minutes left. In that time I would like to explain what I think may be happening and what we are going to do next. Is that all right?

MRS S: Yes, I am anxious to know.

DR D: As you say, your doctor has been treating you as though you have irritable bowel, but you have not responded to treatment and you have begun to lose weight and bleed. The first thing we need to do is to check just what is happening with your bowel by doing some X-rays and blood tests.

MRS S: Yes. Do you think it could be cancer?

DR D: Given what happened to your father and the nature of your symptoms that is a possibility. We are not going to know until we have done the tests. So it is important we get on with the tests as soon as possible.

MRS S: Yes.

DR D: Is there anything else you would like to know at this point?

MRS S: No, I just want you to get on with the tests so I know where I am.

It is important that you finish this interview in a specific manner by saying, for example, 'In that case I think we should finish at this point, is that all right?' You should also aim to keep within the time parameters that you negotiated. This educates the patient to make proper use of your time, rather than believing they can always achieve an extension of the time available by leaving important disclosures to the last minute. If you give in to this ploy you will have less time to give your subsequent patients. This is manifestly unfair, as it is your responsibility to ration time equally between patients. How you decide the nature and amount of information that the patient is ready to be given will be discussed in the next chapter.

SUMMARY

Taking care to explain to the patient the aims of the interview, negotiating the time available and note-taking all increase the likelihood that they will disclose their key problems. If you then use the specific interviewing behaviours that are known to promote disclosure, and avoid inhibitory behaviours, the majority of patients will disclose most if not all of their current problems. If you allow time to summarize the patient's problems and check whether any concerns have not yet been mentioned, this will minimize the risk that any key problems remain undisclosed.

REFERENCES

Bensing, J.M. and Sluijs, E.M. 1985: Evaluation of a training course for general practitioners. *Social Science and Medicine* **20**, 737–44.

Goldberg, D., Steele, J.J., Johnston, A. and Smith, C. 1982: Ability of primary care physicians to make accurate ratings of psychiatric symptoms. *Archives of General Psychiatry* **39**, 829–33.

Goldberg, D.P., Jenkins, L., Miller, T. and Faragher, E.B. 1993: The ability of trainee general practitioners to identify psychological distress among their patients. *Psychological Medicine* **23**, 185–93.

Maguire, P., Faulkner, A., Booth, K., Elliotyt, C. and Hillier, V. 1996: Helping cancer patients disclose their concerns. *European Journal of Cancer* **32A**, 78–81.

Stewart, M.A. 1995: Effective physician–patient communication and health outcomes: a review. *Canadian Medical Association Journal* **152**, 1423–33.

Thompson, J.A. and Anderson, J.L. 1982: Patient preferences and the bedside manner. *Medical Education* **16**, 17–21.

chapter 4

GIVING INFORMATION

INTRODUCTION

The two previous chapters have emphasized that effective treatment depends on the doctor's ability to identify the patient's presenting problems and concerns, and the impact of these on their family and daily life. It is also vital that the doctor is able to give information and advice about their patient's illness, treatment and prognosis in a way which ensures that they understand what is being said, remember it accurately and act appropriately.

If the patient perceives that they have been given information which is adequate for their needs, and they feel supported and understood, they are much more likely to comply with the advice and active treatment (Stewart, 1995).

OBJECTIVES

The objectives of this chapter are to describe and illustrate interviewing strategies which will allow you to:

- determine the amount and nature of the information that the patient wishes to be given;
- provide explanations so that accurate understanding and recall by the patient is maximized;
- frame explanations that show an understanding of the patient's own views of what is wrong;
- achieve a shared understanding of the problem and involve the patient in planning what should be done;
- use this information-giving phase of the interview to foster a trusting and supportive doctor–patient relationship.

Before these objectives are considered, some problems with information-giving in practice need to be considered.

PROBLEMS WITH INFORMATION-GIVING

The objectives outlined above are achieved infrequently in practice because insufficient attention is devoted to the information-giving phase. Experienced doctors tend to use a rigid style of information-giving and make assumptions about what patients want to know. This fails to do justice to the extent to which patients vary in their wishes for information about diagnosis, treatment and prognosis. Most doctors assume that patients want information about the offered treatments and likely adverse side-effects and complications. In reality, most patients want information about their diagnosis, possible causes and problems, and the prognosis (Meredith *et al.*, 1996).

Direct observation of doctor–patient consultations has shown that doctors often use medical jargon which the patient does not understand, and they do not ensure that the patient has understood the information being offered. It is not surprising, therefore, that on average patients recall only 50% of the information offered. Only about 50% of patients who are prescribed drugs take them as advised, and even fewer follow advice about changes in behaviour such as diet or level of exercise.

PERFORMANCE OF YOUNG DOCTORS

In one study, 40 young doctors each interviewed 3 patients to elicit their problems. After they had been given the results of the physical examination, investigation, diagnosis and prognosis, they returned to discuss these with each patient, and were given 10 minutes in which to do this. These discussions were recorded on video tape and evaluated. Most of the young doctors gave simple information on diagnosis and treatment, but only a few mentioned investigations, possible causation or prognosis. Moreover, only a minority obtained and took into account in their information-giving the patients' views or expectations (Maguire *et al.*, 1996).

Their poor performance was disturbing. Few of these doctors used a systematic approach to giving information and advice. Most of them began with the data given to them, rather than with a recapitulation of the problems they had elicited or with an explanation that they were moving into the information-giving phase of the consultation. The doctors performed most poorly on the techniques that have been found to improve patient satisfaction and compliance with medical advice and treatment, namely tailoring the advice given by the doctor to the patient's view of what is wrong and their prior expectations of treatment, and checking that information about diagnosis and treatment has been understood and accepted.

There was little discussion of patients' responses to the information and advice given. The reluctance of these doctors to discover the patients' views of their predicament paralleled their tendency to avoid asking about psychological and social aspects in the information-eliciting part of the interview. These problems are not surprising, given that none of these young doctors had been trained in information-giving skills during their undergraduate education.

KEY TASKS

DETERMINING WHAT A PATIENT WANTS TO KNOW

This should be done in four steps.

- Check the patient's perception of what is wrong, and any prior experience
- Check how much information to give
- Check whether the patient has any other information needs
- Recap information needs and check the patient's understanding

Check the patient's perception of what is wrong, and any prior experience

Once you have elicited all of the patient's problems, it is important to recap in order to check that the problems have been correctly understood before you introduce the information-giving part of the interview.

For example, a doctor started by recapping as follows: 'You say you have been passing water frequently, and have felt thirsty and tired. Have you had any thoughts about what these symptoms might be due to?' The patient replied by saying that she thought she had diabetes. The doctor responded by stating that she could be right, but he would need to examine her first and then test her urine. There were no abnormal findings on physical examination, but the urine tested positive for sugar.

The doctor next explained that there was some sugar in the urine, and said he thought it might be diabetes but he would need to do more tests. Before going further, he checked whether the patient had any experience of diabetes in other people. She revealed that her father had suffered from diabetes and needed insulin to control it. Unfortunately, he complied poorly with treatment and developed severe complications, including gangrene in his left leg. Consequently, he had had to have his foot amputated. Shortly after surgery he had a stroke and died.

The doctor responded with empathy by saying 'So, telling you that it is probably diabetes can't be easy for you to bear'. The patient responded by saying that she had always worried that she might get diabetes like her father, but she was hopeful that something could be done for her as she intended to comply with any advice offered.

Check how much information to give

You should then ask the patient whether they would like any other information ('Would you like to know about the tests I would like to do to confirm the diagnosis and the stage of your diabetes?').

Check whether the patient has any other information needs

When you have explained the tests and checked that the patient understands exactly what needs to be done, and after having mentioned a suitable time frame, you should next check whether there is any further information the patient would like ('Is there anything else you would like to ask me?'). This will often provoke questions about the extent to which the illness can be cured or controlled. It is important to screen again after that to check whether there are any further questions the patient would like answered before you give information and advice.

Recap information needs and check the patient's understanding

You should then recap what you believe the patient wishes to know: 'So, you would like to know what tests I wish to carry out and what they will involve, you want to know – if the diabetes is confirmed – whether or not we are going to be able to control it and prevent the kinds of complications your father suffered from, and what treatments might be involved, and you say you have no other questions you would like to ask me, is that right?'

You should then ask the patient to put these questions in order of priority so that you can start with the most important one first.

It is important that you check the patient's understanding by asking 'Can you now tell me what you understand about what I have explained to you in terms of the tests needed, the extent to which we should be able to control your illness, and the likely treatment?'

OPTIMIZING RECALL AND UNDERSTANDING

- Follow a logical sequence
- Break down the information offered into distinct categories
- Use concise language and avoid medical jargon

You should be trying to present information in a way that will maximize the likelihood that the patient will recall accurately what was said and have a proper understanding of it. The extent to which you give information about investigations, possible diagnoses, treatment, complications and prognosis depends on how certain you are about the diagnosis. It is important that you follow a logical sequence.

Follow a logical sequence

Start with your thoughts about investigations, and follow on with a discussion about possible diagnoses, treatments, complications and prognosis. The extent to which you go into each of these depends on how certain you are about the diagnosis. In a case of possible recurrent breast cancer you might proceed as follows:

DR B: You had breast cancer first diagnosed exactly a year ago. You now tell me you have got this severe persistent pain in your right hip which is getting worse. You have said that you are terrified this means your cancer is back. But we also know you have osteo-arthritis in your right hip and that otherwise you have been well in

Mrs J: yourself. So I don't want to jump to conclusions. The first thing we need to do is to check what is going on in your hip by doing some more X-rays. Is that all right?

Mrs J: I hoped that was what you would say because I am very worried that my cancer could be back, and I am finding the uncertainty very difficult.

Dr B: I will arrange for you to have scans as soon as possible. Once the results are back I will get you in to see me straight away. We can then discuss the findings, and what the implications might be for you – is that all right?

Mrs J: Yes, thank you.

Break down the information offered into distinct categories

When the doctor diagnosed asthma in a male patient he proceeded to confirm that the patient's perceptions of what was wrong were correct ('You are right, it has turned out to be asthma').

He then rightly checked how the patient felt about this. The patient responded by saying that he was not worried so long as the doctor felt he was likely to be able to control it. He admitted he was relieved it was asthma because his GP had insisted it was down to 'nerves'. He had not believed his GP even though he was under stress at the time because he was being threatened with redundancy.

In view of the patient's predominant concern, the doctor confirmed that it was very likely that his asthma could be controlled, and he then negotiated with the patient as to how he would like to proceed by giving different categories of information. He therefore said 'What I would like to do, as long as you agree, is to first explain the nature of your asthma, how we might treat it (including the benefits and disadvantages of the treatment), and finally I would like to discuss how you are likely to get on in the short term and in the longer term. Is it OK then if we do it in that order?' The doctor then provided relevant information about the nature of asthma as an illness, and checked that the patient had understood what had been said before he negotiated to move on ('Is it OK now to move on to what we can do in the way of treatment, or do you have any other questions about your asthma?'). When offering information in these discrete categories the doctor should emphasize key points that the patient needs to remember. In this case, the doctor said, in relation to prognosis, 'Bearing in mind your concern about your asthma being controlled, I am hopeful that we can keep it under good control with appropriate medication').

Use concise language and avoid medical jargon

You should provide information in simple language and avoid using medical jargon. If jargon is used, the patient may be reluctant to ask the doctor what was meant by the words. They may therefore leave the consultation with serious misunderstandings about what is wrong with them. Some patients welcome visual information in the form of diagrams or written information and instructions, but others do not. Thus it is important that you negotiate as follows: 'Would it help if I gave you this information in the form of a booklet, diagram or in some other way?' In some instances this might include the provision of audio or video tapes. You should not impose such aids to understanding on patients who do not want them. Some patients do not wish to be reminded of the details of their disease or prognosis, especially if the prognosis is poor.

ACHIEVING A JOINT UNDERSTANDING

You should ensure that you and your patient have a mutually agreed understanding of the patient's predicament and the action that needs to be taken. It is important that this includes an explicit acknowledgement of the patient's view of what might be wrong, and of the treatments offered.

DR A: You said that you thought this pain in your chest was angina because
          of your experience of heart trouble in your brother and father. I can
          also understand why you have been frightened this could mean you
          might die of a heart attack. However, I do not think you have angina.
          I think it is much more likely that the symptoms you have got are
          due to 'heartburn', given what you have said about them and the
          factors that bring it on.
MRS J: Thank goodness. I was terrified it could be angina.

After providing such an explanation, it is important to invite the patient to contribute actively to the dialogue by giving him or her an opportunity to ask questions, seek clarification or express any doubts about what has been said, even if the response seems as clear-cut and positive as in Mrs J's case. Thus you might ask 'Does what I have said leave you with any questions? Was there anything you feel I haven't covered?' This makes it legitimate for the patient to ask questions and voice doubts, and it minimizes the likelihood that they will have continuing concerns about what has been said.

However well you tailor information to what patients signal they wish to know, they may become angry, irritated or distressed. You should acknowledge and explore this, as is shown in the following example.

DR S: As I have explained, you have a severe disc problem. You need
          regular sessions with a physiotherapist over the next few weeks.
MR L: (looking distressed) I am not sure that is possible.
DR S: You seem distressed by what I am saying. Can you bear to tell me
          about it?
MR L: I have only just started a new job. I had been out of work for 2 years.
          My employers are very strict about people taking time off. If I don't
          work our financial problems will get even worse. Isn't there some
          other way of sorting out my disc problem?

When patients don't give obvious signals of their reactions to what has been said, you should ask them directly. For example, in this case, 'Now you have heard that you have a severe disc problem and you need physiotherapy, how does that leave you feeling?'

PLANNING FUTURE ACTION

Whether you are at the stage of deciding investigations or planning treatment you should share your thoughts. This will be perceived by patients as involving them, and it should lead them to feel more satisfied with the consultation and to comply with the advice offered.

DR P: We both agree that you have become severely depressed in the last 6 months following the unexpected death of your mother. You have admitted that you have not been able to grieve because it is too painful. My thoughts are therefore that we should proceed in two ways. First, we should treat the depression with appropriate medication to reverse the chemical change that is causing the depression. Secondly, I would like to help you with your unresolved grief by talking to you about it, especially your feelings. How do you feel about that?

MRS D: I was afraid I was going out of my mind with the depression. I know I need help. I am relieved you seem to understand what I have been going through and some help is available. I am not sure though that I will be able to talk about my mother because I find it so upsetting. We were so close and she was always there to turn to.

DR P: I can understand you are worried that it might be too painful to talk about her death. What I need to do now is discuss how we should proceed. Since your depression is making you feel so negative, I think we should concentrate on alleviating that by giving you specific medication which we call antidepressants. Once you begin to feel less depressed we should try and help you talk about your bereavement, Is that acceptable?

MRS D: Yes, I know I need to feel less depressed before I can face talking about my mother.

When you share your thoughts with the patient in this way it may become clear that the patient is not happy about what is being suggested. You should explore the reasons for the patient's unease about your suggestions, and take these into account when discussing possible alternatives. If the patient rejects advice about a preferred treatment option but you believe that this option is the correct one, it is important that you share your concern and make predictions about the consequences without being confrontative or aggressive. Thus you might say 'I can understand you are reluctant to take medication at this point. However, I don't think your stomach pain is going to going to get any easier without it. In fact I think it is going to get worse. What I would like to do is to review you in 2 weeks' time to see if that is the case, and to see if you will reconsider your views about medication'.

When you offer medication it is important, as with any treatment option, to discuss the benefits and disadvantages and to check whether the patient has understood these, to ascertain their views of the treatment and to establish whether there might be barriers to the patient accepting your advice.

DR N:	There is no doubt you have become seriously depressed since you learned you have bowel cancer. The stress of knowing you had cancer triggered a chemical change in your brain. Your brain is not producing as much of the right chemicals as it should. I would therefore like to prescribe antidepressant medication to try and reverse it. Is that acceptable?
MR M:	I am not very happy about that.
DR N:	Why are you not happy?
MR M:	Aren't they just tranquillizers I will get dependent on?
DR N:	Are there any other reasons you are unhappy about taking medication?
MR M:	Won't they simply act as a 'happy pill', and when I stop them I will be back to square one.
DR N:	If I can take your first point about them being tranquillizers, they are *not* tranquillisers, they react differently. They reverse the chemical disturbance which is the basis of your depression and will enable you to get back to being the person you were before. Nor do they act as an artificial stimulant. Are you prepared to consider taking them?
MR M:	Yes.
DR N:	Then I need to explain exactly what drug I would like to use in your case, and what the possible side-effects might be.

When offering treatment options it is important to check whether the patient has someone they can turn to and by whom they will feel supported. Thus, in the above example, the doctor might have asked 'How do you think your wife will feel about you going on medication?' The patient might reply 'She was very keen I got some help with this problem. I am sure she will be supportive'.

When explaining the investigations, the doctor should check whether the patient understands exactly what is involved, and also whether they have had any previous experience of such investigations in themselves or a key relative. Otherwise, major concerns about the investigation may be missed and lead to unnecessary anxiety and distress, and even avoidance of the investigations.

DR B:	As we have discussed, your symptoms are due to angina. Given your strong family history of heart disease, we now need to check the state of your coronary arteries by doing an angiogram. Do you know what that is?

Mr R:	It involves putting some dye into my blood vessels and seeing through some kind of X-rays what is going on in my heart, but I am scared of it.
Dr B:	What scares you?
Mr R:	Being put under. I am terrified I won't come round afterwards.
Dr B:	Why is that?
Mr R:	When I had a hernia operation 2 years ago it took me a day or more to come round, and they said I was sensitive to the anaesthetic.
Dr B:	Shall we talk to the anaesthetist together about these fears?

The doctor should be honest about the possible adverse side-effects of the investigation, and should ascertain whether the patient is willing to accept these. They should also inform the patient of the relative merits of the investigation and its advantages. The patient should then be asked if he or she has any further questions about what is proposed.

OFFERING CHOICE

Sometimes there are genuine treatment choices available to the patient – for example, active intervention versus a wait-and-see policy. The relative merits of each treatment option should be discussed openly with the patient if this is their wish. They should then be asked if they wish to be involved in the choice or if they would prefer to leave it to you. A substantial minority of patients prefer to leave the choice of options to the doctor, but the remainder adjust much better psychologically if they feel they have been involved in the choice. If a choice is not possible you should explain why that is the case.

If patients feel that they have not had a choice, but they had a strong preference, they are more at risk of not adapting well psychologically. For example, a woman developed profound body image problems following a mastectomy for treatment of her breast cancer. She could not look at herself without becoming very distressed. She would not allow her husband to look at her, and she started wearing clothes that concealed her shape. She was especially angry because she had been originally told she had to have a mastectomy. She then found out that because her disease was diagnosed early and her lymph nodes were not involved, she could have had a wide local excision followed by radiotherapy. She consequently felt cheated and found it more difficult to come to terms with the loss of a breast than she might perhaps otherwise have done.

ADVISING CHANGES IN BEHAVIOUR

Sometimes a key aspect of management is that you have to advise the patient to make changes in their lifestyle – for example, reducing their cigarette, alcohol or food consumption. The nature of their lifestyle, their beliefs about it, their cultural background and their attitudes to trying to change their behaviour, in terms of the perceived benefits and outcomes, should first be explored. The extent to which they feel confident about their ability to change their habits (self-efficacy) should be assessed, as well as their views of the likely outcome of their efforts (outcome expectancy). Effective change is unlikely to occur if there is evidence of low self-efficacy and negative outcome expectancy.

The patient needs to be confronted openly with the need for change and the problems that will arise if they do not make such changes. Their readiness for change should be checked to establish whether they are merely thinking of change, are willing to take active steps to help to secure that change, or have already considered what steps are needed and are taking these.

SUMMARY

When you make efforts to establish your patients' views of their predicament, you should show that you have taken these into account and have made an effort to find out exactly what information the patients want, be responsive to their reactions to the information given and, where appropriate, involve patients in decision-making and choice. It is likely that they will then feel satisfied and comply with the advice and treatment offered, and that they will feel supported and cared for.

REFERENCES

Maguire, P., Booth, K., Elliott, C. and Jones, B. 1996: Helping health professionals involved in cancer care acquire key skills – the impact of workshops. *European Journal of Cancer* **32A**, 1486–8.

Meredith, C., Symonds, P., Webster, L. *et al.* 1996: Information needs of cancer patients in West Scotland: cross-sectional survey of patients' views. *British Medical Journal* **313**, 724–6.

Stewart, M. 1995: Effective physician–patient communication and health outcomes: a review. *Canadian Medical Association Journal* **152**, 1423–33.

chapter 5

INTERVIEWING KEY RELATIVES

INTRODUCTION

The provision of effective support by key relatives makes a major difference to how patients adjust to their illness and treatment. It minimizes unnecessary use of health services, improves compliance with advice and treatment offered, and can mean that patients are able to continue to cope at home instead of being admitted to hospital. This fosters the patient's psychological adjustment and reduces the risk that they may develop anxiety or depression (Baider *et al.*, 1996).

OBJECTIVES

This chapter will describe:

- the key elements of support;
- the factors that affect relatives' ability to provide support.

It will also highlight:

- specific communication problems within families;
- strategies for assessing relatives' adjustment;
- how to deal with difficult problems within families, including:
    denial;
    collusion;
    differential coping;
    skewed relationships;
    family conflict;
    demanding relatives;
    talking to children;
    complaining relatives.

Finally, it will discuss the impact of culture on family adjustment.

KEY ELEMENTS OF SUPPORT

- Practical support
- Accepting and coping with role changes
- Coping with relationship changes
- Being able to discuss concerns
- Realistic attitude

PRACTICAL SUPPORT

It is important that patients feel they can obtain practical support from their family and friends when it is needed. For example, they may need help with transport in order to get to and from their general practitioner or hospital. If they have young children or elderly infirm relatives, they may need help looking after them while they are absent.

ACCEPTING AND COPING WITH ROLE CHANGES

Longer-term illnesses and treatments demand significant changes in roles within the family because the patient becomes too ill or disabled to carry out their normal chores within the home. They will feel well supported when these role changes are accepted by their relatives without argument.

For example, when a man developed severe coronary heart disease he was advised to stop working and to 'take life easy'. He was the breadwinner of the family and only 45 years of age. His wife dealt with the situation by discussing it fully with him and finding a job so that there was a regular income coming into the home. She did this willingly and this took a huge burden off the patient. Their two children were now grown up, and she felt that she was making a positive contribution to the situation.

COPING WITH RELATIONSHIP CHANGES

Because of the stress of disability in major illness, patients may go through periods of being unhappy and irritable. They will feel supported if their loved ones understand their reactions and are not judgemental about them. Illness and disability may also affect their sexual drive and activity. Again, if they perceive that the partner, for example, is accepting these changes and not falsely attributing them to a negative change in their emotional relationship, they will derive great support from this.

BEING ABLE TO DISCUSS CONCERNS

A major source of support is for patients to feel that they can discuss their concerns about their predicament openly with close relatives and friends, and that they will be understood by them.

REALISTIC ATTITUDE

Most patients have a realistic attitude to the likely outcome of their disability or illness. They will feel most supported if their relatives have a similar realistic attitude, rather than adopting an unnecessarily positive or negative view of what is going to happen in the longer term.

Although such support from key relatives is most important in fostering patients' psychological adjustment to their situation, the relatives will only be able to provide that support if they are able to cope with the demands of the illness and its treatment. Therefore the factors that affect relatives' ability to cope merit discussion.

FACTORS THAT AFFECT RELATIVES' ABILITY TO PROVIDE SUPPORT

The following factors will be considered:

- Perception of support
- Time out from caring
- Coping with role changes
- Satisfaction with medical information
- Patients' psychological adjustment
- Denial or unrealistic expectations
- Collusion
- Differential coping
- Skewed relationship
- Conflict about telling children
- Need for careful assessment

PERCEPTION OF SUPPORT

Relatives need to feel supported both practically and emotionally by their other relatives and friends. They also need to know that the patient and others involved understand their predicament and the demands being placed on them. They need to have confidence that other relatives and friends will help them with any difficulties, and that their general practitioner and employer will be particularly understanding.

For example, a man had to take his wife for chemotherapy on a regular basis for 1 year. Consequently, he had to take time off work frequently to take her for treatment, but his employer complained about this. Although he knew the circumstances he threatened the man with the loss of his job, saying that he would find someone to replace him who did not have to take time off. Despite this threat he could find no-one else who could take his wife to her chemotherapy appointments. He also felt that he should accompany her because of her distress about the treatment and worry about her prognosis. His wife also experienced quite severe side-effects with the treatment, and this made his dilemma in his own words 'almost intolerable'. He developed signs and symptoms of a depressive illness and required help for this.

TIME OUT FROM CARING

Some illnesses and disabilities mean that relatives are faced with a major burden of care – for example, if they have to look after a patient who has dementia or who has become bedridden. It is important that they have opportunities for time out and respite, otherwise they will be gradually overcome by the practical and emotional burden of coping with the patient. If they are involved in caring for the patient during the last few weeks of life, they may be left with unpleasant images of the nature of their illness and suffering. They may have exhausted their emotional and physical energy, so that when they finally experience a bereavement they cannot cope with the loss. Relatives tend to believe that it is their duty to cope, and that they must be seen to be doing so. They also tend to regard the care of the patient as the key priority, and assume that they therefore have no right to disclose the burden they are experiencing both physically and mentally. Often when asked directly how they are coping, they will pretend there are no problems. Consequently it is all too easy for doctors to underestimate the real burden on key relatives and the adverse effects that this may be having on their health.

COPING WITH ROLE CHANGES

If relatives are resentful about having to change their role within the family (for example, taking on much more responsibility for looking after the children) and these role changes persist, they are at much higher risk of becoming emotionally distressed themselves, and even of becoming anxious or depressed, than relatives who are able to accept the role changes involved.

SATISFACTION WITH MEDICAL INFORMATION

When relatives feel satisfied with the information they are receiving from doctors about the patient's condition and prognosis, they will feel much more confident about what is happening, and better able to provide support.

PATIENTS' PSYCHOLOGICAL ADJUSTMENT

About 25–30% of patients with chronic disabling or serious life-threatening illness will develop clinical anxiety or depression. These disorders can result in the patient becoming very irritable, despairing and difficult to reassure. This can alienate their relative, who does not understand why they are behaving in this way, and it may prevent them from being as supportive as they could be. It can also lead to them finding the situation so difficult that they themselves become anxious or depressed.

DENIAL OR UNREALISTIC EXPECTATIONS

Some relatives will not accept the reality of the patient's predicament, and will insist that there is nothing seriously wrong with him or her even though they have been told that the illness is incurable. Such relatives will often have wholly unrealistic expectations about the effect of treatment. They can become very demanding about what they expect from the medical profession, and be difficult to cope with. Because they do not accept the patient's reality, they will not be willing to listen to his or her concerns and respond appropriately.

COLLUSION

Collusion is said to occur when the relatives genuinely believe that the patient cannot cope with the truth about his or her situation. They therefore insist that the patient should not be told the diagnosis, as they fear that on hearing this they will turn their head to the wall, give up and die. When the relatives take this position they are placed in a terrible dilemma. They are unable to discuss with the patient the most important thing that is happening to him or her and themselves. They can also feel under increasing strain because they know they are lying to the person they love. This prevents the patient receiving support, but it also carries a high risk that the relatives themselves will not receive support if the other people around them disagree profoundly with their behaviour. This can lead to increasing friction and conflict.

DIFFERENTIAL COPING

There can be major differences of opinion among close relatives with regard to how open they should be about what is happening. For example, a woman who had multiple sclerosis preferred to be open about it and about risks of further deterioration. She had a realistic view of what might happen in the future, and was neither too pessimistic nor too hopeful. However, her husband found it extremely painful to have her talk about it, and would insist that she changed the subject. This made her very angry, and she felt that he did not care about her. However, it was because he cared so much about her that facing the reality of the likely course of her illness was too painful for him to contemplate. He felt increasingly isolated from his wife and unable to provide support.

SKEWED RELATIONSHIP

A skewed relationship is said to have developed when the bond between a patient with a serious disability or illness and a particular relative becomes so strong that it excludes the rest of the family, who then feel disfranchised and unable to provide support.

For example, a family of four were coping well until a 13-year-old son developed leukaemia. After a stormy illness and many complications, he died 3 years later. His mother became seriously depressed and required psychiatric treatment.

She was extremely bitter about his death and kept asking 'Why him, why me, why has he been taken from me?'

It became clear that he had been a very special child to her. Before he was born she considered that she was happily married and related well to her husband and 3-year-old daughter. When her son was born he was especially loving and cuddly, and he also developed a strong sense of humour. Because of this she found him good company and became increasingly close to him emotionally. She started to feel that he was the only one in the family who gave her enjoyment and love.

When he was diagnosed with leukaemia she found this very difficult to accept. She became involved in his treatment, and this was intensified by pressure from nursing staff for her to take over a lot of his daily care. His treatment required frequent out-patient visits and in-patient admissions. She was always present and consequently became even more involved with and close to him. Consequently, she had increasingly less time for her husband and daughter, who began to feel disfranchised and abandoned by her. By the time the boy died, the relationships within the family had deteriorated seriously. She felt wholly unsupported by them, even though they had done their best to help her. Her perceptions at the time of the death were that she was the only one who had cared for the boy, and the others were being selfish.

CONFLICT ABOUT TELLING CHILDREN

There can also be major conflict when a parent is seriously ill and it has to be decided whether the children should be told anything about the situation or how much information they should be given.

NEED FOR CAREFUL ASSESSMENT

If relatives are to be helped to provide support for the patient and to avoid problems themselves, you must be able to assess how they are coping with the patient's illness and treatment, and whether they need help in their own right. You also need to be competent in managing the situations that preclude effective support, as discussed above.

ASSESSING RELATIVES

The main aims of assessment of relatives are:

- to elicit the relative's account of the patient's problems;
- to elicit their perceptions of diagnosis and treatment;
- to ascertain the impact on their ability to cope on a daily basis, and on their mood and key relationships;
- to elicit any other key problems;
- to check their information needs, adjustment to role changes, patient's adjustment and level of coping.

Assessing relatives together or alone

The first decision you must make is whether relatives should be interviewed separately from the patient. Whenever possible you should see them separately because relatives will usually withhold their major concerns out of fear of distressing the patient. You should therefore be explicit about your need to see them alone. For example, you might say ' I have had a chance to talk with you now about your problems. You say I have a reasonable understanding of what has been going on. It would help me now if I could talk to your husband about his view of what has been happening to you. Is that all right?' Most patients accept this so long as you add that once you have seen the relative, you will then see the patient and the relative together.

Content to be covered

You should seek first of all to ask the relatives to give a history of the patient's presenting problems in their own words. You can then check whether this is consistent with the patient's account ('Can we start by asking you to tell me what you have noticed has been wrong with your wife in recent months?'). At this stage it is also important to check the relative's perceptions directly ('Given all that has been happening, what do you make of what's going on with your wife at the moment?'). The relatives should then be asked how they have been affected in themselves ('Can you bear to tell me how all this has been affecting you yourself?'). If the relatives' responses do not include comments on how their daily life, mood or relationships have been affected, direct questions should be asked ('Just how has all of this affected your ability to cope day to day? How has your mood been? Have you at any time felt particularly low and anxious? Has it affected your relationship with your wife in any way? How have the rest of the family been affected?'). This educates the relatives that it is legitimate for them to disclose their own concerns about their own reactions, rather than to continue to believe they should only talk about the patient's illness and reactions. The doctor should then screen to check whether the relative has any other concerns ('In addition to what we have talked about, are there any other concerns you have about what is going on?'), and check how they feel about key factors that may affect their ability to support the patient, unless these have already been volunteered.

Satisfaction with medical information

'How do you feel about the information you have been given to date about your wife's condition and treatment?'

Role change

'You mention that you are now having to do all the housework in addition to your own job. How do you feel about that?'

Relationship changes

'You say that your wife has lost all interest in sex and has asked you to sleep in a separate bed for the time being. How are you feeling about that?'

Coping methods

'Are you able to discuss what is happening together or not? Why not?'

Such an assessment should also reveal whether there are any problems with the relative being in denial, adopting a policy of collusion, coping differently to the patient, establishing a skewed relationship or having conflicts about openness. If any problems become apparent, you must explore their exact nature and extent, particularly if they concern conflicts within the family or problems in negotiating important role changes.

Finally, it is important to double-check whether the relatives have any other concerns that have not been disclosed ('Do you have any other concerns about the situation you would like to mention? Are you sure?'). It can be difficult for the relative to decide on the spur of the moment what these other concerns might be. It is therefore helpful if you suggest, for example, 'Perhaps you would like to have some time to think this over and let me know if you would like to talk again about things'.

If differences in coping are present, it is important to ask the relatives what they think about the patient's way of coping compared to their own method, to see if they can tolerate it and are respectful of it, rather than becoming angry and bitter.

MANAGING KEY PROBLEMS

Key problems you may encounter are:

- Denial
- Dealing with collusion
- Differential coping
- Skewed relationships
- Conflict between relatives
- Demanding relatives
- Telling children
- Complaining relatives
- Families from different cultures

DENIAL

Denial will usually be evident from the relatives' response to your question about what they believe is wrong with the patient. It might present as unrealistic demands for treatment which you know will not be successful. They should be confronted in a constructive way with the reality of the patient's illness. Thus, in response to a statement from a relative that she cannot understand why you are not doing more to help her mother, you might say 'Realistically I am afraid she is not responding to chemotherapy. We hoped there would be a response but there hasn't been any. Unfortunately, we are not able to give her any more chemotherapy. We have tried all that is available'. The relative may retaliate by insisting that there must be other treatments. It is important that you confront them with the reality that this is not the case ('I wish there was another option. Unfortunately there isn't in her case'). It is then important for you to be empathic ('I appreciate it must be hard for you to accept this is the end of the line. I wish other treatments could be offered, but it is simply not the case'). The relative may insist that there must be other centres that could offer help. It is important to confront the relative again with the reality that this is not so ('Unfortunately, I don't think there are. You are welcome to get a second opinion but I don't honestly think it is going to result in any further treatment. It must be hard for you to realize that this is the end of the line'). The relative will usually accept the situation at this point and the approach to be followed is the same as that discussed under bad news in Chapter 6.

If a relative still appears to be in denial and, for example, insists his wife is going to recover, he should be challenged in two ways. First, the inconsistencies should be raised, given the fact that she has deteriorated and failed to respond to treatment ('You insist she is going to get better, but you admit she has lost more weight and has been complaining of increasing tiredness. I am puzzled that you can reconcile the two'). If this does not work, it is useful to find out whether there is any window on denial by asking 'I know you are hoping your wife is going to get better. May I ask if there is ever any time, whether it is in the waking day or when you are sleeping, that you consider things won't work out?' Many relatives who appear to be completely in denial will admit that they do wonder at times, albeit briefly, if the patient is going to recover. You should then negotiate to see whether they can talk about that reality for a few minutes and discuss the implications. This can allow relatives in denial to move forward towards awareness and begin to adapt to what is happening.

DEALING WITH COLLUSION

Collusion should not happen from an ethical viewpoint. The General Medical Council guidelines, *Duties of a Doctor: Confidentiality*, insist that 'patients are entitled to expect that the information about themselves or others, which a doctor learns during the course of a medical consultation, investigation or treatment, will remain confidential'. Doctors therefore have a duty not to disclose to any third party information about an individual that they have learned in their professional capacity. They are also charged to 'protect all confidential information concerning patients and clients obtained in the course of professional practice and make disclosures only with consent, where required by Order of the Court or where you can justify disclosure in the wider public interest.' Thus collusion should not happen. Unfortunately, it still occurs relatively frequently when relatives insist that the doctor must not tell the patient the truth. The request to collude is usually based on the relative's wish not to face the patient's resultant distress, as well as their love for the patient and a wish to protect them from undue anguish and suffering. It is misguided because it usually has the opposite effect. Patients who are the victims of collusion generally feel increasingly isolated because they realize that major facts are being kept from them. They are also at greater risk of anxiety and depression and problems with symptom control.

When faced with a relative who is colluding, the first step is to explore their reasons for this ('Can you tell me why you believe you shouldn't tell your husband what is going on or have him told by the doctors?'). The relative will usually reply that they cannot bear to upset them further and that the patient will give in and turn 'their face to the wall'. You should not challenge this belief but respect it and say 'You could be right, you have known him a long time'. You should then establish the strengths of those reasons ('Just how strongly do you feel about this?'). This will usually reveal that the relative has genuine and deeply held beliefs about the adverse consequences of the patient knowing the truth. There is no point trying to persuade relatives that they are misguided. Instead, you must enquire whether they have experienced two kinds of cost, the emotional cost of lying to someone they love ('Just how have you been affected during this period since you decided that John shouldn't be told?') and the adverse effect on their relationship ('Just how has it affected your relationship with John?'). These questions usually reveal that there has been a profound and increasing emotional strain, and that a major barrier has been developing between them.

The next step is to summarize the relative's reasons for collusion, acknowledge the costs and ask for permission to talk with the patient to check their awareness (see Chapter 7).

Checking the patient's awareness will usually reveal that they are indeed aware of what is going on. Both the relative and the patient should then be asked if they would like to talk with you in order to work through their resultant concerns. It is important if you meet with, for example, the couple immediately to acknowledge the distress that the shared knowledge is now causing them, and then establish the concerns that are contributing to that distress so that they can be identified and steps taken, where possible, to resolve them.

DIFFERENTIAL COPING

When differential coping is evident it is important to deal with this early on. Although it is preferable to promote openness, this may not be possible because one of the family members finds it too painful to confront. It is important to respect a relative's need to deny the gravity of a patient's illness, and to educate the patient that this denial is a consequence of love and not neglect.

SKEWED RELATIONSHIPS

It can be difficult to correct the skew. For this reason, it is best to try to encourage sharing of the load of care for a sick child, for example, from the early stages of illness. If either parent resists this, their reasons should be explored. It may then become apparent that one of the parents needs to be over-involved, and they should be confronted about this. Perhaps this is best done by one of the senior members of the medical team or a social worker. The risks of the family becoming disfranchised emotionally should be emphasized.

CONFLICT BETWEEN RELATIVES

The needs of the different protagonists should be established by meeting them separately where possible and then arranging a joint meeting. If they insist on continuing to disagree about the patient's management, it may be necessary to call in another member of the team to try to resolve it. You should explore whether such conflict preceded the patient's illness. If it did, it is unlikely that anyone is going to be able to resolve the conflict now without major therapeutic input. It needs to be questioned at the outset whether this is merited. In contrast, if conflict has arisen since the diagnosis of the illness and treatment, then a solution can usually be found.

DEMANDING RELATIVES

Some relatives are very demanding in terms of what they expect to be done for the patient, the level of care given, investigations performed and treatments provided. It is important that the relatives are confronted constructively with regard to what can reasonably be done and what is unreasonable. If their demands continue, it is important to confront them with the fact that their requests are unusual, and the basis of these should be explored. This will normally be due to major fears or guilt. The relatives may know that they have not done their best for the patient, and are now trying to compensate for this by making excessive demands on the hospital. Excessive demands can also arise from their anxiety that the patient might die. If you think this is the case, it is worth reflecting it back as an educated guess: 'As we are talking, I get the feeling that underneath all this you are worried about what might happen to your wife'. If the relatives present their demands in an angry manner, their anger should be acknowledged and the strategies discussed in Chapter 7 should be used.

If their demanding behaviour continues, it is important that you set limits by, for example, saying 'Although I told you we won't know what is happening for a few days, you are ringing me several times a day to check what is happening. If I keep being bleeped to answer the phone calls, I am not going to be able to give my attention to her care as well as that of other patients. So it is important we agree a reasonable frequency of contact by phone over the next few days. Is that all right?'

If the frequent calls continue, you must be willing to adhere to what was agreed in terms of the acceptable frequency of telephone calls.

TELLING CHILDREN

Openness in the family about serious illness in a child is known to promote the psychological adjustment of all family members. Therefore it is important that you encourage openness whenever possible. However, a key issue is when to introduce the fact that a child has a serious and life-threatening illness to the other children. One way is to suggest that relatives ask the children what they understand of what is happening: 'What do you make of what has been happening to Daddy in the last few weeks?' They can then tailor their responses according to how the child responds, as described in the advice on breaking bad news in Chapter 6. If the patient is currently well, it may be better to advise them to postpone any detailed discussion until there is a marked deterioration, and at that time the children can be asked if they have any questions, and these should be answered honestly.

COMPLAINING RELATIVES

This problem may present with a relative being angry, in which case they should be handled as described in the section on handling anger in Chapter 7. When the complainant is calm and rational, you should explore the nature of their complaints, the basis of these and exactly how they feel about it. The relative should then be asked if there is anything else that has made them complain about the care given. Only when all their complaints have been aired should you try to respond to them (in the complainant's order of priority).

When complaints are justified it is important that you apologize and ask the relatives what they would like to be done about it. Most relatives simply want reassurance that the doctor and hospital or general practice will do their best to ensure that the situation does not occur again. They are not looking for an excuse to sue the hospital. Apologizing when complaints are legitimate reduces the risk of litigation rather than increasing it (Levinson *et al.*, 1997). In contrast, being defensive and saying little leaves a vacuum in relatives' minds about what has happened. This serves only to fuel their fears and suspicions and increase the risk of litigation.

When they say they would like to ensure that the problem does not occur again it is important to ask them to be explicit about what steps they would like to be taken. Their requests will usually be reasonable. It is helpful to ask if they would like to hear that something concrete has been achieved in relation to their complaints. It is also important that you make a detailed note of the complaints and the relatives clearly acknowledge that you have understood their complaints before they are processed. A note to that effect should be placed in the case-notes, dated and signed.

FAMILIES FROM DIFFERENT CULTURES

Families from some cultures believe that they should take all of the responsibility for looking after the patient. Their wishes should be respected so long as this does not interfere with the treatment of the patient or become a serious burden to them. If it does, they should be confronted with this in a constructive manner and given the opportunity to choose whether they will continue with their own strategies or be flexible. They may argue that the patient must not on any account be told the truth. This should be dealt with as described above for breaking collusion. It is important to explore the underlying reasons for their beliefs and to respect these, including those beliefs that have a religious or spiritual basis.

SUMMARY

Families play a major role in supporting patients. Any problems that they are experiencing should be actively identified and appropriate action taken to try to resolve them. Otherwise, their ability to provide support as well as their own physical and mental health may be compromised.

REFERENCES

Baider, L., Cooper, C.L. and De-Nour, K.A. 1996: *Cancer and the family*. Chichester: John Wiley & Sons.

Levinson, W., Roter, D.L., Mullooly, J.P., Dull, V.T. and Frankel, R. 1997: Physician–patient communication: the relationship with malpractice claims among primary care physicians and surgeons. *Journal of the American Medical Association* 277, 553–9.

chapter 6

BREAKING BAD NEWS

INTRODUCTION

The way a doctor handles a consultation involving the breaking of bad news can have a profound effect on the later psychological adjustment of patients and relatives.

It has been found that there is a strong relationship between patients' perceptions of the adequacy of the information they were given about their illness and treatment and their longer-term psychological adjustment (Fallowfield *et al.*, 1990). Patients who consider that they were given too much or too little information at the time of diagnosis are at much greater risk of becoming very distressed or developing anxiety and/or depression. Therefore the doctor's first task is to determine what the patient is ready to know, and to avoid imposing information if the patient signals that they do not want it.

When a patient has signalled they are ready to hear bad news and that news has been broken, it is crucial to given them an opportunity to discuss their concerns in detail. These will include those concerns they had before the consultation because they had been worried about their signs and symptoms, and had perhaps heard worrying information when talking with other people. They could also be concerned as a result of hearing the bad news itself. Giving patients the opportunity to discuss their concerns and to mention and express the feelings associated with them has been found to be therapeutic and to result in more manageable levels of distress. Even if their concerns cannot be resolved, most patients feel less distressed if they have been able to voice their concerns and feel that they have been understood by the treating clinician. If concerns remain undisclosed and unresolved, the patient is likely to become depressed and anxious (Parle *et al.*, 1996).

OBJECTIVES

The objectives of this chapter are to describe strategies that will improve doctors' ability to:

- establish patients' awareness of what might be wrong;
- determine how much information to give;
- break bad news so that the risk of overwhelming emotional distress or denial is minimized;
- elicit the patient's concerns and feelings;
- respond to these concerns;
- handle any difficulties that may arise.

CHECKING PATIENTS' AWARENESS

The strategies you should use when breaking bad news will depend on what that patient already knows about the nature and extent of the illness. Therefore the first essential step is to find out what patients know already and how they have been affected by this knowledge. Doctors commonly ask patients 'What have you been told already?' Although it is important to know what has been said to patients by other doctors, it often gives a misleading idea of the patient's actual knowledge. Their knowledge will be based on what doctors have said to them, what they have heard while talking to friends and relatives, and information obtained from the media and the Internet. Thus it is more useful if you first ask, after obtaining a history, 'Have you had any thoughts about what your symptoms/problems might be due to?' Over 80% of patients will reveal that they realize they have a serious illness. You should then check whether they have any other sensible reasons for their conclusion ('Are there any other reasons why you think that?'). A few patients will find it too painful and move into denial ('I am being silly. It is some infection I picked up'). This should be respected, as 5–10% of patients do not want to hear the diagnosis.

It usually becomes clear that most patients' notions are sound and based on good reasons. You are then no longer in a position of breaking bad news. Instead, your task is to confirm that the patient's awareness that their illness is serious or incurable is correct. There is no way you can soften this blow. The moment the patient's belief is confirmed as correct it will be painful. Thus, you might say, for example, 'I am afraid you are right, we are not going to be able to cure your cancer'.

WHEN PATIENTS ARE UNAWARE

It is much more difficult to break bad news when the patient has little or no awareness of the gravity of their situation. For example, a patient had been referred to a surgeon by his general practitioner, and he understood that the most likely explanation for his stomach pains was that he had an ulcer. He had investigations to confirm this, and still strongly believed that his problems were due to a stomach ulcer. When the surgeon asked him what he thought was wrong, he said immediately that he thought he had an ulcer. In this case, the difficult task for the surgeon was how to change the patient's perception from the idea that he had a benign condition to the knowledge that he had a potentially fatal one without provoking overwhelming distress or pushing him into denial. The way he did this was to give a 'warning shot' and then leave space for the patient to signal whether he wished to go further or not. You should only proceed to give more information when the patient gives an unambiguous signal that he or she wishes to know more. This strategy enables you to tailor what you say to what the patient is ready to know.

Leading an unaware patient to a full understanding
You should therefore begin by firing a warning shot that the problem is more serious than the patient has realized. You should then use a hierarchy of

euphemisms from the least to the most obviously serious. This gives the patient time to make the transition from believing their situation is non-threatening to understanding that it is potentially fatal.

DR F: You tell me you have had this gnawing pain in your stomach, your appetite has been poor and you have been feeling sick. What are your own thoughts about what these symptoms might be due to?

MR B: My doctor told me it was an ulcer, and when I first saw you you thought it was, too. He gave me some medication and I felt a lot better for the first few weeks. However, in the last 2 or 3 weeks the pain and sickness have got much worse. But I have been under a lot more stress at work.

DR F: As you know, we hoped it was just an ulcer but I am afraid it is more serious.

MR B: What do you mean? (signalling a wish to learn more about the nature of his problem).

DR F: When we put a tube down to look at your ulcer we took tissue to check what kind of ulcer it was.

MR B: Yes.

DR F: Unfortunately, we found some serious abnormalities.

MR B: Serious abnormalities?

DR F: We found some tumour cells.

MR B: You mean the ulcer is cancer then?

DR F: I am afraid so.

Here the patient made it clear in his response to each of the doctor's statements that he wished to know more. Consequently, the breaking of the bad news could proceed to a confirmation that he had cancer.

PATIENTS WHO ARE AWARE BUT DO NOT WANT ANY MORE INFORMATION

Some patients reveal that they are aware of what is wrong when you check their knowledge of what might be happening. However, they give an explicit signal that they do not wish to be given any more information. It is most important that you respect their wishes.

A woman with cancer of the cervix realized that she had developed a relapse of her disease, and was referred by her general practitioner back to the cancer hospital to consider what further treatment might be given. She made it clear early in the consultation that she realized that her disease had recurred, and said 'I don't want you to give me any detail about what has happened and where it has travelled to, I don't think I could cope with that. I just want to know if you can do anything for me'.

The doctor insisted on telling her that she should be given detailed information about the extent of her disease, for he believed that this was the only way to provide information. He therefore told her that she had recurrent cancer of the cervix which had spread into her pelvis. He insisted on drawing a diagram to show how her disease had progressed. Subsequently she experienced powerful and intrusive images of cancer spreading throughout her body, and she was unable to banish these from her mind. Over the next 24 hours she became agitated and depressed, and was referred for an urgent psychiatric opinion.

PATIENTS WHO ARE UNAWARE AND DO NOT WANT INFORMATION

When asked what they think is happening, up to 10% of patients deny the gravity of their situation and indicate that they do not wish to receive more information. Despite this, they usually ask about possible treatments. Therefore you must not pressure them to confront what is going on, as their denial indicates that it is too emotionally painful for them to do this.

Instead, you should check how solid their denial is. There are two ways of doing this. The first is to challenge them constructively with any major inconsistencies in their history. For example, a young woman insisted that her swollen abdomen was due to a further pregnancy. When the consultant said he was very puzzled that she thought she was pregnant, because her symptoms were different from those of a previous pregnancy, she was able to acknowledge that she realized she had been trying to persuade herself that the situation was not serious. The fact that he mentioned he was puzzled by the inconsistencies between her history and past experience led her to reveal that 'deep down' she knew it must be serious and was probably ovarian cancer. This turned out to be the case.

Some patients who are in denial will not acknowledge such inconsistencies. You should test the waters by asking 'Has there been any time during the waking day or in dreams when you have thought that your illness may be more serious?' Checking if there is a window in their denial in this way may reveal that there are times when the patient has acknowledged that their illness could be serious. If you then negotiate ('Can you bear to talk about this further?'), some patients will acknowledge that they have sometimes thought the illness could be serious, life-threatening or even fatal, and will be prepared to talk more about this. Despite the use of these strategies, some patients still remain in denial. It is important to respect this, as it may be their only way of coping with a difficult situation which would otherwise overwhelm them.

ELICITING PATIENTS' RESPONSES TO BAD NEWS

Once the bad news has been confirmed or broken, doctors tend to feel that they have a duty to help the patient feel there is hope by immediately offering information and reassurance. Thus they leave the patient little time to react to the bad news and voice their concerns about what they have heard.

A major consequence of this lack of enquiry is that the patient's key concerns remain undisclosed and they remain preoccupied with them. Therefore, while the doctor is giving important information about the nature and stage of the illness and the treatment options, the patient is not assimilating this. Instead, their concerns are intensifying, as in the following example.

A surgeon was seeing a 29-year-old woman to break the bad news that she had breast cancer. He knew from a previous consultation that she was already worried that she might have the disease. The tests had confirmed that she had a localized tumour, it had not spread to her lymph nodes, and she would be able to have a lumpectomy followed by radiotherapy. The surgeon believed that she would be relieved that her prognosis was good, so he approached the consultation in a positive frame of mind.

He did not know, because the patient had not felt able to tell him, that her sister had died 6 months ago from breast cancer after a 2-year history. Her sister had been told that her prognosis was good, but she had died quickly. In the last 3 months of her life she had suffered from pain, lost a lot of weight and become bedridden. The patient had nursed her over the last 3 months and had been left with strong recurring and intrusive images about this time period. When the surgeon confirmed that her belief that she might have breast cancer was correct, she immediately connected with these strong images. Because he did not ask her whether she had any concerns about the bad news and what her feelings were, she became increasingly preoccupied with the negative images. As he spoke she was only listening for any negative information that confirmed her right to be pessimistic about her future. When he mentioned 'We will have to give you radiotherapy to mop up any "residual cells"', she concluded that her pessimism was justified and that she would be dead within the next 2 years.

Because her overt levels of distress were not unusual, the surgeon had no idea that she was reacting badly. He came out of the consultation feeling optimistic that she had a good prognosis and would cope well. The reasons for this reluctance to enquire about patients' concerns and reactions after breaking bad news were discussed in Chapter 2.

Therefore, after you have confirmed or broken bad news, you should follow these steps.

After breaking bad news

- Pause and say nothing
- Acknowledge the patient's feelings
- Elicit all of the patients' concerns
- Elicit the patient's feelings
- Prioritize and address each concern
- Pitch advice at a realistic level
- Prioritize other concerns
- Screen for other concerns

ACKNOWLEDGE THE PATIENT'S FEELINGS

Unless you explicitly acknowledge the patient's distress, they will not feel they have permission or space to talk about it. It is therefore important that you signal this by saying, for example, 'I can see that what I have told you has come as a great shock (or confirmed what you thought already). Would you mind telling me just how you are feeling at this point?'

This may seem a banal question to ask someone who has just been given bad news, but it is vital as it gives the patient explicit permission to talk about their concerns and feelings.

The patient may react angrily by saying 'How do you think I am feeling?' It is important that you respond by explaining 'I realize it may sound like a stupid question, but it is most important that I understand just how you are feeling at the moment, because every individual is different'. Most patients will respond helpfully. You should then check (negotiate) whether they are prepared to talk about the reasons, as some patients may find it too painful. A useful question is 'Do you mind telling me what is making you feel so distressed?' If they say it will be too upsetting to do so, this should be accepted. Most patients give important cues about their main worries. Your task is then to elicit their major concerns *before* you offer any advice or reassurance. You should also encourage the patient to mention and express the feelings associated with their concerns.

ELICIT ALL OF THE PATIENT'S CONCERNS

In this example, the doctor has just broken the bad news to a patient that she has had a second recurrence of lymphoma soon after a course of chemotherapy. She is now seeking to elicit all of the patient's concerns and associated feelings:

DR M: I am sorry I have had to tell you that your disease is back again.

MRS H: But I have only just finished the second course of chemotherapy.

DR M: I can see you are very upset (acknowledges emotion). Can you bear to tell me just what concerns you have at this point? (negotiation)

MRS H: I am at the end of my tether. Each time I have had chemotherapy the lymphoma has come back. I have been to hell and back with all the sickness and tiredness. It now seems an utter waste of time.

DR M: I think I can understand how you feel given what you have been through. Can you bear to tell me if you have any particular concerns? (asking about concerns)

MRS H: I can't bear the thought of more chemotherapy. I couldn't go through it again. But my daughter is due to get married next May. I am terrified I won't be alive then if I don't have more treatment.

DR M: So you are concerned about whether you can cope with more chemotherapy, and whether you will be alive to see your daughter married. Before I talk to you about these things can I first check if there is anything else bothering you?

At this point the patient responds angrily – 'Are these not enough problems?' This is a common response, and it is important for the doctor to explain her question ('Yes, but it is important I check whether you have any other concerns so I can help you appropriately').

When eliciting the patients' concerns the doctor should invite her to talk about any related feelings, but she must do so in a negotiating manner, as it could be too painful for the patient to talk about the relevant feelings.

ELICIT THE PATIENT'S FEELINGS

DR M: Can you bear to tell me how all this is leaving you feeling in yourself?

MRS H: I knew my disease was back, but it is so unfair. Why do I have the kind of lymphoma that hasn't responded to chemotherapy? What have I done to deserve that?

DR M: It does seem unfair.

MRS H: It is, especially as my daughter is due to be married soon.

DR M: You mentioned worries about the chemotherapy, and not seeing your daughter married. Which of these would you like to discuss first?

MRS H: Are you going to be able to do anything about the lymphoma? Can you control it for long enough that I can see my daughter married?

By asking the patient how she is feeling about her predicament, the doctor learned that she was very angry that she had a type of lymphoma that did not respond to treatment, particularly as her daughter was due to be married. The doctor also realized that her concerns about further chemotherapy were justified in the light of prior side-effects. When the doctor invited the patient to define her priorities, the main one was whether there was any prospect of treatment for her lymphoma.

It was important for the doctor to summarize the patient's main concerns, because that indicated that her worries had been heeded.

PRIORITIZE AND ADDRESS EACH CONCERN

Time constraints can make it difficult for you to cover all of a patient's concerns within one consultation. It is therefore important to help them to determine which is the most important problem for them to resolve. Other problems can then be left until later. Otherwise, time may be wasted on unimportant concerns, while major issues remain unresolved.

To help the patient to define their priorities, it is important to ask them, after summarizing their concerns, 'Which of these problems would you like to discuss first?' Few patients have difficulty in deciding what they want help with first.

The next task is to give advice about what might be done with regard to each issue of concern.

PITCH ADVICE AT A REALISTIC LEVEL

The doctor explained that she would like to try some different chemotherapy ('I would like to try some new chemotherapy. However, in view of your being so worried about adverse side-effects, I think we should only try one course first to see how you get on, and then we can discuss where we go from there. If you can tolerate it better than the other chemotherapy, we should be able to give you several courses and we may get a worthwhile response.'

This honest bargaining approach allows the patient to buy into what might be upsetting treatments without having to agree to a whole course. Often they tolerate the treatment better than they thought they would, and then accept more treatment and achieve a better treatment response.

PRIORITIZE OTHER CONCERNS

Once the concern about further chemotherapy has been dealt with, the doctor rightly asks the patient which of her other concerns she wishes to discuss next:

MRS H: I am desperate to go to my daughter's wedding, but I am frightened I am not going to live long enough.

DR M: That's an awful position to be in (empathy). The problem is I just don't know. It depends on whether you can tolerate the chemotherapy and get a reasonable response. What I suggest we do is see how you get on. We can then discuss whether you should ask your daughter if she is willing to bring the wedding forward. Would that be all right?

MRS H: I guess it's the only option in the circumstances.

SCREEN FOR OTHER CONCERNS

At this point any doctor could be forgiven for believing that all of the patient's concerns had been elicited. However, it is possible that important concerns have remained undisclosed. It is therefore crucial to ask a screening question ('In addition to what you have mentioned, have you any other concerns?'). More often than not the patient will indicate they haven't, but occasionally such screening questions reveal important undisclosed problems:

DR M: I know we have talked about your worries about chemotherapy and your daughter getting married and your fear of pain. Before we finish, can I just check if there are any other concerns you have not had the chance to mention?

MRS H: I don't know how I am going to cope with my husband.

Faced with this new and unexpected concern, Dr M rightly explores this by asking 'Can you bear to tell me what your concerns are about your husband coping?' The patient replies by saying that he has not been able to talk about her illness since the diagnosis because he finds it too upsetting. She is worried that this lack of communication between them will be intensified now that her disease has recurred and she needs more chemotherapy.

WHEN TIME IS SHORT

It is important that the doctor checks what is the patient's main concern and then explains that the other concerns will be dealt with soon, at a subsequent consultation. Patients are tolerant of this approach provided that they believe the doctor has identified and understood their main concerns. They are not expecting the doctor to 'fix it all' within one consultation. However, they do need to feel that he or she understands what they are worried about and will respond appropriately in due course.

At the end of any bad news consultation, patients who wish to know the reality of their predicament should realize the nature of their situation, but should find that their distress levels are within manageable limits and feel hopeful that something can be done to resolve most if not all of their concerns.

DIFFICULTIES ENCOUNTERED ONCE THE BAD NEWS HAS BEEN BROKEN

DIFFICULT QUESTIONS

When bad news is broken effectively it can prompt difficult questions, such as 'Am I going to die?' You must acknowledge that this is a key question but add that you would first like to check why the patient is asking this question at this point in time. Although most patients want a clear answer, some are testing the waters and are not sure they want to know the truth. At the moment they ask the question they prefer to avoid facing reality and go back into denial. The only way to check this is to reflect the question back to the patient as in the following example:

Ms A: Am I dying?

Dr M: I am going to answer your question, but can you first tell me why you are asking me that just now?

Ms A: You told me my cancer was back and you weren't able to give me any more treatment. I have been feeling increasingly tired and weak. It takes me all my time to get out of bed, and I am so much more breathless.

Dr M: Are there any other reasons why you think this means you are dying?

Ms A: It is exactly what happened to my uncle when he died from lung cancer.

Dr M: I am afraid you are right. We are not going to be able to cure you, and we have no more active treatment.

The doctor then proceeds to acknowledge the patient's distress and asks if she is willing to discuss her concerns.

Sometimes, when patients are invited to reflect on why they are asking that question, they reveal that they do not wish to confront the situation. In the following example, when a patient asked if she was dying the medical oncologist reflected the question back and found out that even asking the question had made her wish to pretend that her illness was something she had picked up in the tropics:

MRS N: Am I dying?

DR M: I will answer you that in a minute, but can I check why you are asking me?

MRS N: Oh, I am just being silly, it's some disease I've picked up in the tropics.

The doctor can double-check that the patient wishes to move back into denial by asking 'Do you really believe this is the case?' In this instance, Mrs N indicated that it was, which indicated that she wished to remain in denial, having come close to confronting the fact that she was dying.

HANDLING UNCERTAINTY

Often you cannot give a patient any certainty about whether or not the disease will respond to treatment. You should acknowledge that the uncertainty is real, empathize with the patient and say 'This uncertainty must be awful for you'. This is reassuring because the patient then knows there is an inherent uncertainty. It allows them to show the doctor how upset they are about this, and the impact it might be having on their daily life.

Patients can then be broadly divided into two groups – those who don't want any more information and those who do.

Patients who don't want any more information

These patients respond to the question 'Would you like any more information?' by saying that they are happy with the information they have been given, but prefer to put concerns about their illness and treatment to the back of their minds. There is no point in imposing further information on them. They will cope well between appointments unless there is some definite physical deterioration. It is therefore appropriate that the doctor next discusses future steps in management and treatment.

Patients who do want more information

These patients should be given as much detail as they wish, including, for example, looking at their scans to see evidence of secondary disease. They should also be asked if they would like markers of symptoms and signs that might herald later deterioration. Follow-up should be negotiated in terms of how long they feel they can cope psychologically before they begin to worry about their situation again. Most patients request follow-up within a 2- to 3-month interval. There is no evidence that patients handled in this way become phobic about their disease. When patients have been given markers of progress it is important to advise them that if they notice any of these markers they should get in touch immediately in order to be reassessed by their doctor.

NEGOTIATING MARKERS

Dr H: Would you like me to tell you what changes might indicate your disease is deteriorating again?

Mr W: That would be helpful.

Dr H: There are several possibilities. At the moment your disease is stable, but if your cancer came back you would probably feel breathless again. You might notice you are losing weight, coughing up blood and feeling pain. If any of these things happen, please get in touch with me. It doesn't matter if it turns out to be nothing. It is better to check you so that if your illness has come back we can try and deal with it. Is that all right?

Mr W: Yes.

Dr H: How long do you think we could leave it before we assess you again, presuming you stay as well as you are feeling now?

Mr W: I think I could manage say 2 to 3 months.

Many patients with advanced disease can maintain a reasonable level of psychological adjustment when their uncertainty is handled in this way and they are offered clear markers.

SUMMARY

First you should check the patient's awareness of the seriousness of their situation, and either confirm that their awareness is correct or fire a warning shot if it is not. You can then use a hierarchy of euphemisms and proceed according to the patient's responses. Once the bad news has been broken, pause to allow a little time for assimilation, then acknowledge the patient's distress and negotiate to elicit their concerns. It is best to elicit all concerns by summarizing and screening ('Are there any other concerns in addition to your pain and exhaustion?'). Encourage the patient to mention and express their associated feelings, and then summarize all of their concerns and ask them to prioritize them and work through them in order of importance.

Avoid premature or false reassurance, check the patient's needs for information and respond accordingly, and if the prognosis is uncertain you should acknowledge this and empathize with them. It is helpful to provide markers for those patients who want them, and to negotiate follow-up intervals.

Always reflect difficult questions back in order to check that the patient is ready to hear an honest answer, and be empathic throughout without being distracted from your task.

REFERENCES

Fallowfield, L.J., Hall, A., Maguire, P. and Baum, M. 1990: Psychological outcomes of different treatment policies in women with early breast cancer. *British Medical Journal* **301**, 375–80.

Parle, M., Jones, B. and Maguire, P. 1996: Maladaptive coping and affective disorders among cancer patients. *Psychological Medicine* **26**, 735–44.

chapter 7

HANDLING DIFFICULT SITUATIONS

INTRODUCTION

However well you try to elicit patients' problems, you may encounter difficulties because the environment in which you are trying to conduct the interview is unsuitable, and there may be severe time constraints. During the course of interviews patients may become very distressed, unhappy or angry, or express feelings of hopelessness. You therefore need to be familiar with strategies that will help you to deal with these situations in an effective but caring way.

OBJECTIVES

The objectives of this chapter are to discuss:

- how to interview in difficult environments;
- how to handle time constraints;
- how to handle strong emotions;
- how to distinguish worry from anxiety and unhappiness from depression;
- how to handle anger;
- how to handle hopelessness.

INTERVIEWING IN DIFFICULT ENVIRONMENTS

Ideally you should assess any new patient, whether they are acutely ill or not, in private. This maximizes the likelihood that the patient will disclose what is troubling them, and will prevent you from being distracted by other events. This can be difficult to achieve in busy environments such as hospital wards and Accident and Emergency departments, where there are often no interviewing rooms available. If you are forced to interview a patient in public, you should try to create as much privacy as possible by the use of screens or curtains. You should check with the patients if this is acceptable, as they may be claustrophobic and unable to tolerate feeling closed in. If they are suffering from a mental illness such as major depression or schizophrenia, they may be experiencing paranoid delusions and worried that you might be about to harm them. Asking the patient if it is all right to draw the curtains or to put a screen around will usually reveal these fears and indicate that they would prefer to be seen in the open cubicle or ward.

When you have to interview patients in such restricted environments you need to be aware that they may withhold important information because they fear it will be overheard by other people. Therefore you must check later whether anything was missed out from the initial history.

RELATIVES WHO INSIST ON BEING PRESENT

Although it is helpful to obtain information from a relative about what has been happening to the patient in order to achieve a more accurate diagnosis of their problems, it is best to obtain this separately and first interview the patient on their own. Otherwise, the patient is likely to withhold information about key problems and concerns because they wish to protect their loved ones from distress.

For example, a woman presented to her general practitioner with complaints of headaches. Her husband insisted on going into the consultation with her. After obtaining a history of her headaches, the general practitioner asked her if there were any other problems. She denied that there were any other difficulties. In reality, however, the couple had been trying to have a child for 10 years but had been unsuccessful. The patient was now terrified that her husband was fed up with this situation and was about to leave her for another woman. She had been feeling increasingly tense and anxious, and this was the basis for her headaches. She was not prepared to admit this in front of her husband, and it only emerged later on a subsequent visit. Thus it is best if you negotiate that it would be more helpful to see the patient alone first and then, provided that the patient agrees, you can see the relative either separately or with the patient. Most relatives accept this arrangement, as they know that they will have access to the doctor soon.

INTERVIEWING WHEN TIME IS SHORT

Because of other demands you may realize that you can spend only 10 to 15 minutes determining a patient's problems. You should advise the patient of this situation and explain that the time will be best spent focusing on the main problems. You should check that this arrangement is acceptable and then explain that you will come back soon to clarify whether there are any other problems.

DR B: I am Dr B, Mr Burns' Senior House Officer. I have been asked to come and see you about this pain you have been getting in your side. Unfortunately, I am in the middle of a clinic and so I've only got 10 or 15 minutes to spend on this occasion. I appreciate that this may not be long enough to cover all the problems you are concerned about. However, I wonder if you would be prepared to tell me what the main problems are that concern you most at the moment. I can then arrange to see you soon to clarify any other problems. Is that all right?

Mr M:	Yes.
Dr B:	I wish I did have more time, but I thought it was better to see you today rather than not at all.
Mr M:	That's all right.
Dr B:	So, what are your main problems at the moment?
Mr M:	It's this awful pain I have been getting in my side.
Dr B:	Would you like to tell me about it?

This honest approach usually gains patients' respect. They understand the constraints on doctors' time and will make every effort to focus on their problems and provide a clear history. If you give no warning that the time available is limited, they will have no idea that they have to disclose their problems quickly. They may not even have disclosed the most important problem before the interview has ended. This can cause patients to feel angry and frustrated because they thought they had more time available to them. Occasionally a patient will respond to your honesty about the limited time available by saying that it is not sufficient and they will only talk when more time is available. You should accept this and negotiate a time when you can give them more time.

HANDLING STRONG EMOTIONS

DISTRESS

Either at the outset of the interview or later on the patient may become very distressed. You should deal with this immediately and constructively, otherwise, they will become preoccupied with the concerns that are provoking their distress, and will cease to concentrate on giving you a history of their current problems. Moreover, their distress is likely to intensify and may become overwhelming.

> You should use the following strategies to handle patient distress:
>
> - Acknowledge the distress
> - Negotiate to explore the reasons for it
> - Screen for other reasons

You should first acknowledge the distress, even though this may seem both unnecessary and banal. You should then negotiate to check whether the patient can bear to explain why they are so distressed, for there is no other way you can establish if discussing the reasons for the distress will be too painful and potentially damaging for the patient, or if they can tolerate talking about it. Once the most obvious reasons for their distress have been disclosed, it is important to check whether there are other factors contributing to it.

DR B: I can see you are very distressed. Can you bear to tell me what is distressing you?

MRS S: This is the third time I have been admitted to hospital in the last 2 months. My husband is finding it more difficult to cope with. I am worried that this may be the last straw for him.

DR B: In what way?

MRS S: He has got ever so depressed. He has stopped going to work and has just been sitting around the house.

DR B: You say that this admission might be the last straw for your husband. Before we talk about that, are there any other reasons why you are distressed?

MRS S: I am scared my stoma is never going to settle down and I am going to continue to get complications.

DR B: Anything else?

MRS S: Even though I keep telling him it was ulcerative colitis he thinks it is cancer and he is going to lose me. I can't get him to see sense.

Here the doctor has established that Mrs S's distress was related to the impact on her husband of her illness and frequent admissions to hospital, and her worry that her stoma was not going to settle. She felt relieved that she had been able to disclose her concerns and became less distressed. She was then able to tell the doctor what had been going wrong with her stoma since her initial surgery.

ACKNOWLEDGING VERBAL CUES

Patients often present their distress in the form of verbal cues early in the interview. For example, while giving a history of physical complaints the patient may say 'I have felt very anxious', 'I have been getting very upset lately, or 'I am worrying about how things are going to work out'. It is important that you acknowledge such cues immediately and negotiate with the patient to check whether they are prepared to talk about them further. This active acknowledgement educates the patient that you are interested in them as a person. It will increase disclosure of their concerns as well as the speed at which they disclose them (Goldberg et al., 1993; Maguire et al., 1996). Even if the cue is not acknowledged immediately, the patient will repeat it. If you ignore cues then the patient is likely to decide that you are not interested, which may lead them to become less disclosing. Therefore if you think you have heard a cue already it is most important that you acknowledge it and negotiate whether the patient is willing to talk about it further.

When picking up and exploring such cues it may become clear that the patient has been anxious, miserable or upset. You then need to establish just how anxious, depressed or upset they have been in order to distinguish normal worry from generalized anxiety disorder and unhappiness and upset from major depressive illness.

DISTINGUISHING BETWEEN NORMAL AND ABNORMAL REACTIONS

WORRY VS ANXIETY

Many patients are worried when they present to doctors for help. In the majority of cases this worry and distress is transient and can be put to the back of their mind. In contrast, morbid anxiety is said to have developed when patients are so worried that, despite their best efforts, they cannot banish their worries. The characteristic features of these worries are that they are intrusive and the patient feels that he or she is being plagued by them.

Generalized anxiety disorder is characterized by the following:

- persistent worry that cannot be banished despite the patient's best efforts;
- persistent worry that occupies over half of the patient's waking time;
- at least four other symptoms of anxiety are present, including:
    irritability;
    difficulty in getting off to sleep;
    impaired concentration;
    feeling tense and on edge;
    tiredness, etc.;
    sweating;
    palpitations.

In the following example the doctor explores how anxious the patient is and whether there are other symptoms of anxiety:

DR D: You say you have been feeling very anxious. Can you bear to tell me more about that?

MR T: Since I got this pain in my chest I have been getting more and more worried that I am going to die from a heart attack.

DR D: Just how worried have you been?

MR T: I can't get it out of my mind, it's with me every minute of the day.

DR D: When these thoughts come into your mind that you might have a heart attack and die, are you able to banish them?

MR T: No, I can't. They just take me over. I don't seem to be able to do anything about them. It's driving me up the wall.

DR D: Just what kind of state of mind do you get into?

MR T: I get very panicky. My heart goes thump, thump, thump and I am frightened it is going to increase the risk of me having a heart attack. I can't stop sweating. I keep shaking. I wasn't like this until I had the chest pains. I find I just can't relax and I get so tense and irritable.

Dr D's further questioning established that the patient had initial insomnia, poor concentration and felt tired on waking. He therefore concluded that this man was suffering from generalised anxiety disorder.

The importance of establishing this is that no amount of reassurance will help this man until his anxiety has been treated appropriately.

In the next example, although the patient was worried, her anxiety was not of morbid degree.

Dr M: You say you are worried this lump might mean your cancer has returned. How worried have you been getting?

Mrs E: It's on my mind quite a lot of the time, but not all the time.

Dr M: Are you able to put it to the back of your mind at all?

Mrs E: Yes, most of the time. It's only when I wash myself, read something in the paper or see something on television about cancer that I start worrying. However, I am hopeful that it will turn out to be nothing.

In this case, despite being in a potentially distressing situation, this woman was able to control her worries and cope normally.

UNHAPPINESS VS DEPRESSION

If during the interview the patient mentions that they have been feeling unhappy, miserable, low or depressed, it is important to check whether they are referring to a normal reaction or to a depressive illness.

Major depressive illness is characterized by the following:

- persistent low mood that the patient cannot banish despite their best efforts;
- low mood that persists over time and occupies over half of the patient's waking day for 2 to 4 weeks;
- a low mood that is perceived as qualitatively and quantitatively different to being merely unhappy;
- at least four other symptoms must be present and/or repeated, including:
    early morning waking;
    irritability;
    impaired concentration or memory loss;
    loss of energy;
    loss of appetite;
    loss of weight;
    loss of libido;
    inability to enjoy life;
    feelings of guilt;
    feelings of hopelessness;
    feelings of pointlessness;

contd

feelings of unworthiness;
feelings of being a burden;
suicidal ideas;
tiredness and fatigability;
social withdrawal.

Characteristically the mood may be worse at a particular time of day, often in the morning. In the next example, Dr M is talking to Mrs C, a patient with severe arthritis which has been causing her considerable pain and major disability. Mrs C discloses that she has been feeling very miserable since finding out that her condition was advanced and unlikely to improve without surgery on her knee.

DR M: You said you have been feeling very low. Can you bear to tell me more about that?

MRS C: The pain is so bad I can only just tolerate it despite the pain killers. What has really got me down is that I am finding it very difficult to get out and about.

DR M: Just how low have you been getting in your mood?

MRS C: Very low.

DR M: What have you been like at your lowest?

MRS C: I get to thinking I have no future. I can't pull myself out of it. I have been so irritable with my husband and children. I'm a burden to them. I'm not able to do what I used to do for them.

DR M: How many days in each week do you feel so low?

MRS C: Every day.

DR M: How much of each day do you feel low?

MRS C: I wake up feeling very low and I don't come round until the evening.

DR M: How does this compare with how you are normally?

MRS C: I was usually the life and soul of the party. Now I can't face going out and talking to people. I won't even answer the phone or go to the door when someone knocks. I am not me any more.

These responses confirmed that Mrs C was suffering from depressed mood and other symptoms of depression, including irritability, feeling a burden, feeling useless, withdrawing socially and feeling worse in the early part of the day.

Open directive questions are often necessary to elicit other important symptoms. These should include questions about sleep: ('How has your sleep pattern been since you started feeling low?', 'Can you describe a typical night?'), loss of concentration ('How has your concentration been? For example, how do you get on when you try to read a paper or watch television?'), loss of interest ('Have you been as interested as usual in things like your hobbies and work?'), loss of energy ('How has your energy been?'), loss of appetite ('Has there been any change in your appetite?'), loss of weight ('Has there been any change in your weight recently?'), social withdrawal ('Have you been seeing as much of people as usual?'), hopelessness ('How do you see things working out?'), worthlessness or uselessness ('How do you feel about yourself as a person?'), feeling a burden ('How do you feel about yourself in relation to others?'), and diurnal variation of mood ('Do you find your mood is worse at any particular time of day?').

When depressed mood is evident you should check whether there is any risk of suicide. This is dealt with in Chapter 9.

HOW FAR SHOULD PATIENTS' EMOTIONS BE EXPLORED?

The aim of exploring patients' emotions or responses is to establish the exact nature and extent of them, and to determine whether or not they represent an abnormal reaction. Even if you consider that you have understood a patient's responses, they may wish to add more. You should check this by summarizing what you have learned and then asking if you have an accurate picture of how they are feeling. When the patient agrees that your picture is accurate, you should negotiate to move on to the next topic. However, if the patient indicates that they do not feel their reactions have been understood, you should give them an opportunity to correct the picture. In the next example the doctor first summarizes his understanding of the impact that the colostomy has had on Mrs P. He then learns that there are other matters which she wishes to disclose:

DR T: So, when you woke up and found you had had a colostomy you say you felt devastated?

MRS P: Yes.

DR T: And you say that you have been worrying about how you were going to manage your bag when you returned home and terrified it might affect your relationship with your husband?

MRS P: Yes, I am frightened he won't be able to accept it and it will put him off me.

DR T: And you say that these feelings are worse when you catch sight of your bag or have to empty it?

MRS P: Yes.

DR T: Do you feel I've got a sufficient understanding of your concerns about your colostomy? If not, is there anything you would like to add?

MRS P: I feel very self-conscious about it. I worry that people will only have to look at me to know I have had a colostomy. I'm worried that it might bulge, leak and smell.

DR T: Any other concerns?

MRS P: No.

DR T: Is it all right then if we now move on and I'll talk about these concerns later and what we might be able to do about them?

If you fail to check with the patient that you have covered their concerns about key events adequately before moving on, the patient may not disclose other important problems. Moreover, when you move the conversation on they will remain preoccupied with the undisclosed concerns and will make less effort to give you an accurate history.

Sometimes patients will say that exploration of their reactions would be too painful and upsetting. This view should be respected.

AVOIDING EXPLORATION BEING TOO UPSETTING

The most important step is to guard against this possibility by negotiating ('Can you bear to talk about this feeling of being "devastated"?'). During dialogues with patients about upsetting matters you should continue to negotiate to ensure that they are still prepared to continue to talk about these issues.

DR J: You say you were devastated by losing a breast. Can you bear to tell me about that?

MRS E: I felt my world had been turned upside down. I no longer felt like a woman. I felt like a freak. I couldn't bear to let my husband look at me. I still can't. I do everything to avoid him catching sight of me.

DR J: Can you bear to tell me why?

MRS E: I am scared he will be disgusted with how I look and that will be the end of our marriage.

A key question here is what Dr J should do next. Should he pause and give Mrs E space to think about her concerns, and hope that she will volunteer further information about her reactions to her mastectomy? Should he be more proactive? Many doctors are taught to just sit and listen when they encounter a situation of this kind. In reality, patients like Mrs E become increasingly preoccupied with their problems and with strong images. In this case, Mrs E will perceive herself as increasingly ugly, unattractive, useless and about to be abandoned, and the images in her head will be like enlarged coloured photographs. Her levels of distress will increase and she will feel more despairing. You can avoid this 'spiralling down' by maintaining momentum in the interview.

MAINTAINING MOMENTUM

You can prevent the patient from spiralling down into even stronger emotions by actively acknowledging their distress as soon as it becomes apparent, and then checking whether there are any other concerns (in this case, about the mastectomy). This questioning has the effect of moving the patient from feeling potentially overwhelmed by their concerns to feeling that they are potentially manageable.

DR J:	Are there any other reasons why you are so distressed?
MRS E:	I am scared he will be disgusted with me and that will be the end of our marriage.
DR J:	No wonder you have felt so devastated, then. Are there any other concerns you have had about losing a breast?
MRS E:	I have felt very self-conscious at work. I felt everybody must know I have lost a breast even though I have not told many people. It has been an effort to go into work. At times I have been tempted to stay at home.
DR J:	Any other concerns?
MRS E:	No.
DR J:	Is it all right if we move on then?

At this point Mrs E felt that the doctor had understood the impact of her mastectomy, and she was ready to move on to another topic. This allowed her to lift herself out of her distress and focus on other issues.

HANDLING ANGER

If a patient is angry at the outset of a consultation or becomes angry during it, it will be tempting for you to become defensive and accuse them of being unreasonable because you feel you have been making a genuine effort to try to understand their problems and to help them. Defensive responses ('We have been doing our best, don't you realize how hard we have been trying to sort it out?') will exacerbate patients' and relatives' anger and make them even more difficult to handle. The strategies you should use will depend on whether the anger is rational, irrational or pathological.

RATIONAL ANGER

As soon as you realize that a patient is angry, you must acknowledge this and invite the patient to explain the reasons for it. All of the causes of the anger should be explored, and defensiveness should be avoided. You should make every effort to identify the intensity of the anger ('Just how angry have you been?'), because this allows the patient to express the anger as well as to talk about the reasons for it. This should result in an obvious defusion of the anger and a transition during which the patient moves from feeling very angry to expressing other emotions such as sadness. In the following example, an initial exploration of the patient's anger suggests that it is due to him having been kept waiting. However, further exploration elicits more profound reasons for the anger.

DR P:	You seem very angry.
MR K:	I am furious.
DR P:	Would you mind telling me what's making you so angry?
MR K:	I have been waiting for 3 hours. My GP told me I would be seen

immediately when I came here, and that my headaches would be sorted out.

Dr P: So, you're angry at having been kept waiting and concerned about your headaches?

Mr K: Yes.

Dr P: Are there any other reasons why you are so angry?

Mr K: My headaches have been getting worse and I have been worried that it might be due to a bleed in my brain.

Dr P: Why do you think that?

Mr K: My brother died of a subarachnoid haemorrhage. He had similar headaches but they were dismissed by his GP as due to stress. He died before he could be got to hospital. I have felt very angry because I felt my headaches were not being taken seriously.

Dr P: No wonder you have been so worried and angry. Can I just check if there are any other reasons?

Mr K: Isn't that enough?

Dr P: Obviously those are a lot of good reasons, but I need to understand if there are any other reasons why you have been angry.

Mr K: There is no other reason.

Dr P: Can you tell me just how angry you have been feeling?

Mr K: I got to the point where I felt I could strangle somebody.

Dr P: I can understand that. I think we need to focus on these headaches of yours so we can work out what might be causing them. Is that all right?

Mr K: Yes.

Because the doctor acknowledged the patient's anger, and explored the reasons for it and the intensity of the anger, Mr K felt much less angry and was able to share his fear that he might be having a subarachnoid haemorrhage. The doctor was not put off by the patient's retort 'Isn't that enough?' Instead, he explained that it was important to check whether there were any other reasons.

If these strategies fail to defuse the anger, you need to consider the possibility that the anger is irrational.

IRRATIONAL ANGER

The key to handling irrational anger is to be vigilant about whether or not the strategies discussed above are resulting in a defusion of the anger. If the anger continues, you must consider that it has an irrational basis, and feed this back to the patient. The patient will then often quickly identify the real source of their anger.

In the next example a patient was very angry at being kept waiting. Attempts to talk about her anger and explore the reason for it made no difference to its intensity. The doctor therefore asked her directly whether there could be other reasons for her becoming so angry. This led to an important disclosure:

DR M:	You seem very angry.
MISS L:	I am furious.
DR M:	Can you bear to tell me why you are so angry?
MISS L:	You are 10 minutes late.
DR M:	Why should that make you so angry?
MISS L:	It means I am not going to get a full appointment with you and I won't have enough time to tell you about my problems. I feel I'm being short-changed.
DR M:	I can understand you feel you are not getting the full amount of time and feel short-changed, but I got held up in the traffic. What I suggest we do is get as far as we can today and then arrange for a further chat later.
MISS L:	That's no good. I came prepared to talk about my problems but the longer I waited in the waiting-room the more I wondered what's the point.
DR M:	Even though I have explained why I was late and asked you why you are so angry, you still seem furious.
MISS L:	I am.
DR M:	You said earlier that you felt you were being short-changed and you are still very angry. Has anything else happened either recently or in the past to make you feel you have been short-changed and so angry?
MISS L:	As I sat there and waited I thought you were never going to come. I felt you had abandoned me.
DR M:	And why should that be?
MISS L:	You are just like my father.
DR M:	Can you bear to tell me what happened to your father?
MISS L:	He dropped dead in front of me when I was six. I felt deserted and abandoned.
DR M:	So my being late triggered the same feelings of being abandoned?
MISS L:	Yes, it did.

At this point Miss L became very distressed. When invited to talk about it she indicated that she had never got over her father's sudden death. He had died at a time when her mother had been admitted to hospital because of severe multiple sclerosis. She felt that she had lost both parents in the space of a week, and had never come to terms with this. Being kept waiting triggered these memories and made her feel that she was being abandoned again. This was why she was furious when the interview started.

Some patients will remain angry despite the use of these additional strategies, and their anger will escalate as you explore the reasons for it sensitively. You should consider that the patient may be suffering from pathological anger if the anger appears to be out of all proportion to any possible reasons. When people are this angry they will not usually respond to reason or persuasion. Therefore you must set firm limits by saying, for example, 'I can't talk to you while you are so angry. We had better terminate the interview at this point. I will then be prepared to see you later if you calm down'. When using this strategy, you should be aware of the likelihood that the pathological anger may be due to the person having a personality disorder, being intolerant of frustration, unable to control their impulses, having problems with alcohol or drug dependence, or suffering from a severe mental illness such as depression or schizophrenia. Rarely, such anger may occur because the patient is suffering from an organic illness such as a brain tumour. Even so, setting limits will normally result in the patient making an effort to control their behaviour and allow the necessary physical or mental state examination to take place. If this fails to work, then sedation may be necessary.

If a patient demonstrates any overt anger towards you or objects and furniture in the interview room, they should be asked immediately to stop doing this, otherwise the interview will have to be terminated. If you are warned beforehand that a patient is very angry, it is best to ensure that you have someone else sitting in with you. Otherwise, such patients should only be interviewed in a room that has a panic button available and where there are staff who can respond quickly if the panic button is pressed.

When confronted by an angry patient:

- avoid being defensive;
- acknowledge the anger;
- check how intense it is;
- explore the reasons for it;
- screen for other reasons.

If the anger does not defuse:

- ask if there could be other current or past experiences provoking the anger.

If the anger escalates:

- set limits or get help;
- consider psychiatric and organic reasons;
- use sedation judiciously.

DISPLACED ANGER

A patient or relative may find it much easier to be angry with you than to confront the person who is responsible for their anger. Thus a relative may arrive on the ward only to learn that the patient has died unexpectedly. They may react by blaming the doctors and nurses for the death and accusing them of negligence. It is most important that the doctor does not try to counter their claims, but explores why they feel so angry. Once they have off-loaded all of their anger about what they perceive to have been negligence on the part of the hospital, they may acknowledge that what they are really angry about is feeling abandoned by the person who has died. They may then begin to express great sadness at their loss and talk about the impact of this.

Displaced anger can also mask underlying guilt. For example, a 65-year-old woman was very angry with her husband's general practitioner when her husband died unexpectedly of a heart attack. Two weeks previously he had complained about severe chest pains. He had been examined thoroughly by the general practitioner, who thought that the cause of the chest pains was angina and arranged an appointment with the specialist. The woman was angry because she believed that if the general practitioner had referred her husband sooner he might still be alive. Exploration of her anger established that she was feeling very guilty. He had complained about chest pains for some time but she had thought he was complaining unnecessarily. She wondered if his death might have been prevented if she had taken his chest pain seriously earlier.

HOPELESSNESS

During an assessment patients may volunteer that they feel hopeless about their predicament, or their non-verbal behaviour may suggest this. It is important that you acknowledge this and avoid giving premature reassurance. Instead, you should explore the reasons why they feel hopeless. It may emerge that hopelessness is a rational response to their situation.

DR M: You say you are feeling hopeless about the future. Can you bear to tell me why you feel hopeless?

MRS B: This is the third time in a year that my cancer has come back. The first two times it came back very soon after finishing chemotherapy. The chemotherapy was very fierce. I don't think I could stand any more. I know I am going to die sooner or later, and I would rather not have any more treatment. I would rather let things take their course.

This patient, a 56-year-old woman with recurrent breast cancer, was appraising her situation realistically. She had a poor prognosis, and the chances of further chemotherapy being of benefit were remote. The challenge for the doctor was to give her some hope. He did this by acknowledging her reality and legitimizing her view of her situation. He then discussed possible treatment alternatives, but in a way that gave her room for manoeuvre:

DR M: In view of what you say, I can understand you are reluctant to have more chemotherapy when there is no guarantee of benefit. There are two options. First, it may be that you would consider having more chemotherapy on a trial basis to see if it is as unpleasant as previous courses. Alternatively, you can decide not to have any treatment. If you do, how do you see things going from here?

Mrs B:	I hope I get some quality of life for a little while, but I am frightened about what happens then.
Dr M:	What frightens you?
Mrs B:	That I would suffer too much.
Dr M:	Can you bear to say more about that?
Mrs B:	My mother died of breast cancer. I had to nurse her in the last 2 months. She wasted away and had terrible pain despite painkillers. Towards the end she couldn't look after herself. I can't bear to think that would happen to me.
Dr M:	So, you had a very unpleasant experience looking after your mother. It is not surprising you are fearful about similar things happening to you. But I hope we could be more effective in helping with any symptoms like pain, and trying to help you with nutrition.

This patient decided not to have chemotherapy, but she felt reassured that the doctor would do his best to help her with any symptoms that might arise.

SUMMARY

It is important that you try to ensure that you can assess the patient in privacy. If not, you should negotiate with them about whether they are willing to accept physical and time constraints. Acknowledging strong emotions, negotiating to explore them further, and then exploring them as well as identifying the reasons for them makes all the difference between the risk of these emotions becoming overwhelming and the patient getting back in control. You should try to distinguish anxiety from worry and depression from unhappiness. Anger can be best handled by avoiding being defensive, and by acknowledging and exploring the intensity and the reasons for the anger. If anger fails to diffuse, it is important to invite the patient to reflect on whether there are reasons that might account for this. In the case of pathological anger it is important to set limits and deal with any overriding priority, whether it is medical or psychiatric in nature.

REFERENCES

Goldberg, D.P., Jenkins, L., Miller, T. and Faragher, E.B. 1993: The ability of trainee general practitioners to identify psychological distress among their patients. *Psychological Medicine* **23**, 185–93.

Maguire, P., Faulkner, A., Booth, K., Elliott, C. and Hillier, V. 1996: Helping cancer patients disclose their concerns. *European Journal of Cancer* **32A**, 78–81.

chapter 8

TALKING TO WITHDRAWN PATIENTS

INTRODUCTION

Patients who appear very reluctant to give a history of their current complaints or to explain how they are feeling after major treatments like surgery can be very frustrating to deal with unless you understand the common reasons for withdrawn behaviour and are aware of the strategies that can be used to overcome such reticence.

OBJECTIVES

The objectives of this chapter are to discuss:

- common reasons for patients being withdrawn;
- how to respond to patients according to the reason for their withdrawal.

COMMON REASONS FOR WITHDRAWN BEHAVIOUR

Reasons for withdrawn behaviour include the following.

- Personality
- Anger
- Hidden fears
- Collusion
- Feelings of guilt
- Protecting the health professional
- Shame and humiliation
- Depression
- Paranoid ideas and delusions
- Confusional state
- Psychotic illness

PERSONALITY

Some patients are extremely shy and introverted by nature. They find it painful and embarrassing to disclose much about themselves, especially more personal matters. Giving a history of their problems can therefore be difficult for them. Such shyness and introversion will usually be obvious at the outset of the interview because the patient will try to avoid eye contact and will appear embarrassed. They may also show other signs of discomfort, such as blushing or stammering.

ANGER

Some patients may be feeling very angry because they believe there was a serious delay in diagnosis. Consequently, they may enter the consultation with a high level of distrust and wonder whether it is worth giving their story again because the same errors may occur. Alternatively, they may be angry that they have a life-threatening illness or degenerative disorder which they feel they do not deserve. They may be asking themselves questions like 'why me?' and 'why now?' They realize that their prognosis is poor and that little can be done practically to eradicate their disease. This may lead them to believe that there is no point in talking, because this will make no difference to the progression of their disease. Patients may also be reluctant to talk if they feel that they are victims of false reassurance.

For example, a woman who had a recurrence of multiple sclerosis was reassured it would be temporary and that she would soon be well. However, her relapse persisted and she deteriorated markedly. She eventually reached the point where she felt there was no point in discussing her symptoms with anyone because they would simply belittle them and continue to insist she would recover.

HIDDEN FEARS

Many patients sense that they have a potentially serious condition. However, they may be ambivalent about confronting the reality because it may be too painful for them emotionally – talking might force them to admit the gravity of their situation, whereas not talking about it protects them from confronting it. As long as they avoid talking about their symptoms and concerns they can continue to persuade themselves that they are not as ill as they sense they are.

COLLUSION

It is unethical to give relatives information about a patient's condition without first informing the patient and obtaining their consent. Even so, collusion – where the relatives insist that a doctor withholds the truth from the patient on the grounds that if they are told the patient will give up and die even sooner – still occurs frequently. Patients who are the victims of such collusion become increasingly isolated from their family and loved ones. Although they usually realize what is going on, they do not feel able to share this, and they therefore believe that no one is interested in their views or feelings. For this reason they feel there is little point in saying anything about their situation.

FEELINGS OF GUILT

Some patients have always put other people's needs in front of their own. When such individuals become ill, they feel that they are not entitled to receive as much help as other patients and should not take up the health professionals' time because it could be devoted to helping other people. At the outset of the interview they tend to say that they do not have any problems and therefore do not need help. They are particularly likely to do this if you appear to be busy and under pressure. They believe that other patients' needs are much greater than their own, and worry that they will be a burden to you and your staff.

PROTECTING THE HEALTH PROFESSIONAL

As was mentioned in Chapter 2, when patients have grown to like and respect doctors, they may become more reluctant to disclose important concerns because they do not wish to distress them. Thus patients who are experiencing severe side-effects may be reluctant to admit this because they know that the doctor was keen to give treatment, and they do not wish him or her to know that it is causing such havoc. Similarly, some patients are reluctant to share their fears (for example, that they are going to die) because they are worried that the doctor caring for them may be distressed at hearing their fears. This wish to protect the doctor parallels the way in which the patient protects relatives from their true worries out of fear of causing undue distress.

SHAME AND HUMILIATION

Some patients regard their problems as pathetic, and believe they should have coped better. They worry that they will be judged as neurotic, ungrateful or unco-operative if they say how difficult they are finding it to cope. For example, a patient in a hospice had been a member of a famous army regiment – the Welsh Guards – and he had been proud to wear the uniform. After leaving the army he maintained the same high personal standards. Unfortunately, he developed cancer of the rectum which did not respond to treatment. His disease progressed rapidly and caused a fistula between his bowel and his lower abdomen. Consequently, he had no control over the discharge of faeces on to the surface of his abdomen. He became deeply ashamed of this and insisted that he position himself in a bed close to the toilet. He refused the strong advice from the staff that he should wear his normal clothes, and he was terrified he would not get to the toilet in time when his fistula leaked. However, he did not feel able to disclose this worry to the nursing or medical staff, because he felt he should have been able to cope with it better. He became seriously withdrawn and unwilling to talk to the staff.

DEPRESSION

Patients with a major depressive illness can, as discussed in Chapter 7, feel so low and despairing that they believe everything is hopeless, nothing can be done to help them, and so there is no point in discussing their problems. They may also feel apathetic and find the act of talking too much of an effort. They tend to claim at the outset of the interview that they have nothing to say. Some depressed patients also have strong feelings of guilt and believe that their illness is some kind of punishment and that they are not entitled to be helped. Feeling worthless as a person and also feeling a burden leads depressed patients to avoid making any demands on doctors' time.

PARANOID IDEAS AND DELUSIONS

Some patients fear that the doctor is out to harm them even when they are meeting with him or her for the first time. For example, one patient was reluctant to talk because he believed the doctor was a member of a national organization called 'The Code'. For many years he had been afraid that this organization was out to kill him, and that he must not divulge any information that could be used against him. He was therefore terrified of saying anything to the doctor who was taking a history. In other patients it is distrust of the doctor rather than an actual delusion that leads them to be reluctant to talk.

CONFUSIONAL STATE

Some patients may find it difficult to talk because they have developed an organic confusional state. There will usually be evidence that they have a poor attention span, are easily distractible and may be frightened and agitated. They find it difficult to concentrate and register what you are saying to them, and they appear labile in mood and emotional.

PSYCHOTIC ILLNESS

Patients may become withdrawn because they have developed a psychotic illness and are having abnormal experiences in relation to their thinking, beliefs and perceptions. They may appear distractible because they are hearing voices talking to them or seeing things that are not apparent to the doctor. When they are distracted they may behave inappropriately by laughing or talking aloud as if they are having a conversation. This is because they are in fact having a conversation with the voices they are hearing. They may be afraid to disclose the awful experiences they are having in case the doctor judges them to be mad. The voices may also be actively instructing the patient not to talk to anyone else, and may be threatening the patient that if they talk some dire consequence will follow. Since psychotic illness is often associated with difficulty in thinking, another reason for these patients' withdrawal may be that they cannot put their words together in a logical order. Instead, their speech may appear disconnected and take the form of strands of speech which have little logical connection to each other.

STRATEGIES FOR DEALING WITH WITHDRAWN BEHAVIOUR

INITIAL APPROACH

As soon as it becomes apparent that you are finding it difficult to establish a useful dialogue with a patient, you should acknowledge this in a way that involves the patient and is not judgmental. Thus you might say 'I get the feeling that we are finding it difficult to get into a discussion about your problems.' You should pause to give the patient a chance to respond. Most withdrawn patients will acknowledge that they are indeed finding it difficult to get into conversation. You should then ask why they are finding it difficult. It is important to do this by using negotiation ('Can you bear to tell me just why you are finding it so difficult to talk just now?'). The patient will usually give explicit verbal cues such as 'There is no point', 'It is a waste of time', 'I just can't be bothered, I feel so depressed', 'I don't deserve to have any help', 'I am very frightened' or 'I feel so ashamed'. You should pick up such verbal cues immediately by saying, for example, 'You say there is no point – would you mind explaining what you mean?' The patient may respond by saying 'I know there is no more treatment for my cancer, so what's the use of talking? It's not going to solve that, is it?'

Not all patients respond with helpful verbal responses. Instead, they may give non-verbal cues and may appear increasingly frightened or ill at ease. This is likely if the patient is experiencing psychotic illness, has paranoid beliefs or is extremely shy. In such cases you should acknowledge the non-verbal behaviours immediately and say 'You seem to be getting more frightened as we talk, can you bear to say what is happening?' The patient may then say 'I am not sure I can trust you. Are you a member of the Code?' When you then ask this man why he is asking if you are a member of the Code, he may explain that the 'Code' has been out to destroy him for 20 years. He is worried that they have had access to hospital staff and have brainwashed you into joining a plot to harm him. Further questioning will then establish that he is suffering from a schizophrenic illness.

Sometimes these approaches do not succeed in persuading the patient to talk. You should acknowledge this by saying for example, 'I can see it is too difficult for you at the moment to say anything about your problems, can I come back tomorrow and check how you are? Is that all right?'

Once these initial strategies have been tried, you will need to vary your response according to the reasons for the withdrawn behaviour.

USEFUL STRATEGIES

Personality

If the withdrawn behaviour is due to the patient's personality, you should acknowledge that it is a legitimate difficulty for them and invite them to do their best ('I can understand then why you are finding it difficult to talk with me about your problems. However, it is important that you try to tell me what is going on.

If at any stage you find it too painful and embarrassing, tell me and I'll stop'). If the patient is of a naturally distrusting disposition, it is worth saying 'In that case you will find it difficult to trust me as well. What I suggest we do is start talking about your problems. If at any stage you feel I am not listening properly or understanding please tell me and I'll try and get it right'.

Anger

As discussed in Chapter 7, you should acknowledge the anger and ask patients if they can bear to say why they are angry and explore the reasons for this before trying to take any systematic history. If this reveals good reasons for the anger, you should say 'I can understand now why you have been feeling so angry. No wonder you are finding it difficult to trust me. Can I begin by asking you some key questions about your present problems?' The patient will then normally allow the history-taking process to begin. If you are alert to what the patient says, acknowledge and explore key cues and adopt the active listening techniques discussed in Chapter 3, the patient will begin to sense that you are interested in them. As a result, they will probably start to disclose more.

If an angry patient indicates that he does not want to talk because it is a waste of time as it will not cure him, you should acknowledge this by saying, for example, 'Yes, you are right. Talking with you will not alter the fact that we have no more active treatments for your AIDS. However, you may have some major concerns about what is happening to you, and we might be able to do something about some of those at least'. Most patients will accept such an invitation and reveal concerns that need attention, whether these are physical, psychological, social or spiritual in nature.

If the patient has been the victim of false reassurance you might say 'It may be hard for you to believe what I say in view of what has happened to you in the past. But once we have all the results to hand I have no intention of misleading you about what is going on'.

Hidden fears

If your initial exploration of why a patient is finding it difficult to talk confirms that it is due to a fear of what they may have to face, you should confront their ambivalence 'I can understand that you have considered talking to me because you have to talk about things you are worried about. But I recognize you may prefer not to talk about them so you don't have to think about them. I have to work with the part of you that is willing to try and confront your problems so that I can see if we can do anything about them. On that basis, are you prepared to tell me what has been going on?' Most patients will then try to overcome their ambivalence and talk about what is concerning them.

MR P: I had an attack of MS (multiple sclerosis) 4 years ago. It affected my vision and I found it hard to walk. I was terrified I'd be completely disabled and useless. But over a period of 3 months I made a good recovery. Now my symptoms are coming back and I am frightened of what that means. I find it very distressing to talk about them.

DR J: Given you were frightened of being completely disabled, I am not surprised you find it distressing to talk about your symptoms coming back. Can you bear to say exactly what frightens you?

MR P: It has been affecting my sex drive this time. I can't get an erection and my wife feels I am losing interest in her. I have just got a new job and can't afford any time off. But I feel wiped out. I can't use my fingers properly to work the computer keyboard.

DR J: I can understand then why you are worried. What I need to do is take a careful history of the changes you have noticed and then examine you. We can then discuss what the implications might be and whether we need to do any tests. Is that all right?

MR P: Yes.

Collusion

You should be empathic about the predicament of the victim of collusion and say, for example, 'It must have been hard for you to feel your family did not feel able to tell you what was going on, even though they may have had good reasons for that. I am really interested in what your own views are about what has been going on. Could you begin by telling me what you have made of your illness and treatment to date?' This will usually reveal that the patient has worked out what is going on and is aware that they are suffering from a life-threatening illness. It is then important that the patient's awareness is shared with the family.

Guilt

If the patient has shown feelings of guilt about being a burden, you should explore the reasons why they believe they should not take up any time, and then explain that they are just as deserving of help as other people. It is important to emphasize that it is most important for them to tell you what is really going on, otherwise you will be unable to help them.

Protecting the health professional

If the patient explains their reluctance to talk on the basis that they can see you are too busy and/or they do not want to bother you with their worries, it is important that you educate them that you do have time available despite appearances to the contrary, and that it is important that they say what their main problems are ('I know you are worried that I am so busy and you don't wish to burden me, but I need to emphasize that we have 20 minutes at our disposal if we need it. I would like to focus on what your current problems are, whatever they may be'). Using the proactive methods advocated in Chapter 4, such as asking open directive questions about the patient's perceptions and feelings, and clarifying their responses, educates them that you genuinely wish to understand their suffering and distress.

DR M: You say you are reluctant to say much about your problems because you feel I haven't enough time to understand. Can I explain that we have 20 minutes at our disposal if we need it? I would very much like to focus on what your current problems are and your concerns. If there isn't enough time, I will arrange to see you again soon. So, can you tell me what your main problems are?

MR C: I am afraid I am just being a nuisance.

DR M: Why do you say that?

MR C: My GP tells me I am just being stupid.

DR M: I won't know that unless you are prepared to tell me what is going on. So, can you tell me what the main problems are?

MR C: I have been getting bad chest pains. They grip me here (points to centre of chest). It's like being crushed by a vice. It scares the hell out of me.

DR M: Can you bear to say more about that?

MR C: I am convinced I am going to drop dead from a heart attack.

DR M: Why?

MR C: All the men in my family have done – my father and two brothers. I am the only one left. They all died in their early fifties. I feel I am living on borrowed time and I can die at any time.

DR M: No wonder you feel scared. What I need to do first is find out more about these pains, and then I can examine you and we can talk about what tests might be needed. Is that all right?

Shame and humiliation

If the patient reveals that they do not want to talk because it will humiliate them, it is important that you acknowledge how painful that might be by saying, for example, 'In view of what you say, I can understand it may be difficult for you to tell me what is going wrong, given that you feel ashamed about it. However, it sounds as though whatever it is, it has been very distressing. You might find it easier to share it than keep it secret. On the other hand, if you really don't want to talk about it, that's all right. I am not going to force you'.

DR L: You say that it will be too humiliating for you to talk about what's distressing you, but clearly something is. I cannot help you unless you are willing to tell me what it is, but I realize that you are finding it difficult. Yet you might feel easier in yourself if you could actually bring yourself to share what you find humiliating.

MR W: I find it very hard to talk about. But over the last few months I have been finding it harder to get an erection. I find I just can't manage and my wife is getting fed up with me. She thinks I must have another woman.

DR L: How long have you had this problem?

MR W: Since I had a colostomy. I am terrified that when we are making love it will touch my wife and she will feel repelled. She says she won't but I am worried she will. As soon as I think about this, any hope of an erection goes.

Depression

If depressed patients claim that they are too tired and apathetic to talk, it is important to encourage them to make an effort. Most depressed patients will make an effort to give a history provided that you say, for example, 'I know it is difficult for you, but it is important that you make an effort to tell me what you have been going through'. It is then important to check whether the criteria for making a diagnosis of depressive illness are present (see Chapter 7).

If the patient is expressing feelings of pointlessness, it is important to acknowledge this but to advise that they try and give a history ('I know you say things seem pointless and that nothing can be done to help you feel less miserable. I can't be sure about that unless you are willing to talk to me and let me know just what has been happening to you. It may be that, despite your fears, we can then do something about this problem').

Confusional state

The first step is for you to confirm that the patient is suffering from a confusional state by checking their orientation with regard to time, place and date, assessing their short-term memory by giving them a name and address to remember and checking their recall immediately, 2 and 5 minutes later, and finally giving the serial sevens test in which you ask the patient to subtract 7 from 100 and keep subtracting 7 from the number obtained. You should also ask them whether they are having any abnormal experiences (checking for illusions, misinterpretations and hallucinations), and whether there is any evidence of false beliefs such as paranoid fears that the staff are intending to harm them.

Once you have confirmed the diagnosis, it is important to give the patient a clear explanation of their confusional state and to reassure them that this is the reason why they are having abnormal experiences. It is important to explain that efforts will be made to check why they have developed a confusional state, and meanwhile they will be nursed in a quiet, well-lit room with staff regularly attending to them. While the causes are being investigated it is important to prescribe sedation to help them with their confusion. Drugs such as haloperidol, thioridizine and ativan are usually effective.

It is crucial to establish common causes of confusion quickly.

Causes of confusion include:

- drugs which the patient is taking;
- drug and alcohol abuse;
- chest and urinary infections;
- cardiovascular disorders;
- biochemical electrolyte disturbance;
- trauma to the brain;
- organic brain disease.

It is important to obtain advice from a senior colleague or psychiatrist at an early stage, because the behaviour of such confused patients can become very disturbed and difficult to manage.

Psychotic illness and paranoid ideas

Most doctors feel apprehensive when confronting a patient who is behaving strangely and appears to be out of touch with reality. They are often worried that the patient may be aggressive. However, such patients usually settle well when they realize that the doctor is attempting to elicit and understand their abnormal experiences. Therefore it is crucial that you pick up and respond to any verbal or non-verbal cues that are given about such abnormal experiences. In the next example, a patient with schizophrenia is being interviewed by a medical student who has been asked to clerk him in after his admission.

MISS J: You kindly agreed to talk to me about why you have come into hospital, but I notice as we are talking that you keep being distracted. Can you bear to tell me what is happening to you?

MR D: It's the voices, they keep talking to me. They are telling me I must not tell you our secrets. Otherwise I will be in trouble.

MISS J: You say voices – what exactly are you experiencing?

MR D: Can't you hear them?

MISS J: No, but tell me more about them.

MR D: They are coming from somewhere in this room.

MISS J: Do you know whose voices they are?

MR D: My parents.

MISS J: But your parents aren't here at the moment.

MR D: But I can still hear their voices. They are very clear.

MISS J: Can you tell me what they are saying?

MR D: They are telling me not to tell you our secrets.

MISS J: Can you bear to tell me what secrets you are talking about?

MR D: I believe I am Dr Child. I am really the son of the Queen but no one wants to admit it. My parents will get into trouble if I talk about it.

MISS J: Are there any other reasons apart from your parents that you believe you are the Queen's son?

MR D: When she appears on television I feel she is talking to me and telling me I am her son.

MISS J: How strongly do you believe that?

MR D: I am certain. I keep writing to her at the Palace, but I get no reply.

MISS J: Have you been having any other experiences that have concerned you?

MR D: No.

In another example, the patient looked very perplexed and the doctor responded appropriately.

MISS L: I can't think straight. My thoughts seem scrambled.

DR S: What exactly are you experiencing at the moment?

MISS L: I start thinking about something then I just lose it, it goes, it's so frustrating, it feels like somebody is stealing my thoughts.

If the patient complains of hearing voices or of disorder of their stream of thoughts, it is worth checking for other symptoms of schizophrenia such as thought withdrawal ('Do you feel that people are taking your thoughts away at any time?') thought insertion ('Do you feel that people are putting thoughts into your mind'?), or thought broadcasting ('Do you believe people know exactly what you are thinking and that you can't keep your thoughts secret from anybody else?'). Such psychotic symptoms can be experienced by the patient as tormenting and very distressing. Therefore you must check their impact and, if appropriate, establish whether there is any risk of suicide. Thus when Dr L asked a schizophrenic patient to describe the impact on her of voices which were telling her she was a slag and a whore, she responded: 'I can't take any more, I am at the end of my tether. I have to escape these voices'. Dr L then explored what she meant by escape, and she responded by saying that she was thinking of killing herself. In such cases, the doctor must then assess the risk of suicide as discussed in Chapter 9 and take appropriate action. Failure to clarify such obvious cues when the patient is disturbed can have disastrous consequences.

DR P: You say you are worried you might have a brain tumour because you have been having bad headaches recently. You also say you have been feeling confused. On examination I cannot find anything wrong in your head, but I can see you are very anxious. I will let your GP know and suggest he gives you some diazepam.

In the above example, if Dr P had bothered to clarify what the patient meant by 'feeling confused', a different story would have emerged. The patient would have explained that by 'confused' he meant that he was bewildered about what was happening at home. He had strong feelings that his mother was not his real mother now, but an impostor who had been put there to kill him, and that his real mother had been kidnapped. When he went home he became convinced that his mother was an impostor and would kill him. That night he returned home and killed her. This example demonstrates that it is imperative, when doctors encounter patients with psychotic illness who explain that they are tormented and/or might be at risk of causing harm, that a psychiatric opinion is urgently requested.

SUMMARY

If you are faced with a withdrawn patient, it can be tempting to dismiss them as difficult and to move on to help those patients who are more co-operative.

However, this will only increase the first patient's level of withdrawal and reluctance to talk.

It is important to remember that in most cases there are good reasons why patients become withdrawn. If you acknowledge the difficulty you are experiencing in getting into conversation, invite the patient to explain why it is difficult, and then explore the resulting cues, it is more likely than not that you will establish an effective dialogue with the patient.

chapter 9

INTERVIEWING POTENTIALLY SUICIDAL PATIENTS

INTRODUCTION

Patients who develop chronic illnesses which cause much suffering and increasing disability, and which threaten further physical deterioration and/or a risk of death, are at greater risk of committing suicide than people without such illnesses. It is therefore important that doctors who are looking after physically ill patients are competent at assessing suicidal risk and knowing when a psychiatric referral is indicated.

Approximately 100 000 patients present to Accident and Emergency Departments each year within the UK having taken an overdose or made some other attempt to harm themselves. Nearly half of these attempts will have involved taking drugs such as paracetamol. One in 10 patients will have attempted to harm themselves in other ways (for example, by cutting themselves). Thus it is crucial for doctors to be able to assess whether such patients are at risk of suicide, and to know when to summon psychiatric help. Many National Health Trusts adopt the policy of insisting that such patients have a formal psychiatric assessment, whether by a specialist liaison psychiatry nurse or a psychiatrist. However, every doctor needs to be alert to the risk of suicide and know how to assess this risk. About 90% of people who have committed suicide suffered from a diagnosable psychiatric illness which was either not recognized or was treated inadequately.

OBJECTIVES

The objectives of this chapter are to describe:

- the psychiatric disorders that are associated with an increased suicidal risk;
- how you can assess these disorders;
- the factors that increase the risk of suicide;
- how to assess risk;
- what steps you should take to prevent patients from harming themselves.

MAJOR PSYCHIATRIC DISORDERS ASSOCIATED WITH INCREASED SUICIDAL RISK

The following psychiatric disorders are associated with increased risk of suicide.

- Major depressive illness
- Schizophrenia
- Alcohol and substance abuse
- Generalized anxiety and panic disorders
- Personality disorders

MAJOR DEPRESSIVE ILLNESS

The diagnosis of depression was discussed in Chapter 7. If the patient is depressed it is vital that you assess whether there are features in their mental state which suggest they are at risk of suicide. You should check whether they have negative ideas about the future or other people, how they feel about their health and about themselves as individuals, and whether they have any particular concerns or apprehensions. Thus you should ask 'How do you see the future?' This will reveal whether the patient has feelings of hopelessness or pointlessness. You should also ask 'How do you feel about your relationship with other people?' Feeling that one is a burden to others increases the risk of suicide. The patient should be questioned about how they perceive their health, as people who envisage that they will experience intolerable mental or physical suffering may see suicide as the only solution. They should be asked how they perceive themselves as individuals to check whether there is any evidence of feelings of unworthiness and uselessness. Such an enquiry may also reveal that the patient feels guilty and believes they have no right to continue living. When they are asked if they have any particular apprehensions about the future, this may reveal that they fear some terrible misfortune will occur such as personal bankruptcy, a second holocaust, or the loss of their family in an accident. If they feel that they are a burden to their family they may come to believe, albeit wrongly, that their family would be better off without them.

Patients who have been bereaved recently and have become clinically depressed may find the torment of their loss and the depression too much to handle. This may lead them to consider killing themselves in order to escape from the suffering. They may also believe that suicide will enable them to join their loved ones.

It is therefore important to explore whether the following major mental state features of depression, which are linked to an increased risk of suicide, are present.

> Major mental state features of depression, linked to increased risk of suicide
>
> - Pointlessness
> - Hopelessness
> - Guilt
> - Being a burden
> - Feeling worthless
> - Believing that others will be better off without one
> - Unable to envisage any future
> - Preoccupied with fears of major incurable illness
> - Preoccupied with fears of further suffering
> - Wishing to escape the torment of recent bereavement
> - Wishing to escape the suffering due to depression

One of the best predictors of risk is how a patient makes you feel during an assessment. If you find that you are feeling low during the interview, this is an important clinical sign and should be followed up by appropriate questioning.

SCHIZOPHRENIA

Patients with schizophrenia are at risk for several reasons. They may find their psychotic experiences such as hearing voices or having delusions that they will be harmed so unpleasant and tormenting that they believe suicide is the only escape.

If you suspect that the patient might be suffering from schizophrenia, it is important to invite them to talk about their psychotic experiences ('Can you describe exactly what happens when you hear the voices? What effect do they have on you?'). The risk of suicide is increased if the voices are abusive and accusatory, or if they instruct the patient to commit suicide ('You know you are a slag, you deserve to die, you should go to a motorway bridge and jump off').

It is crucial that you check just how tormented the patient feels by these experiences, and whether they have considered ending their life to escape the torment.

DR T:	You say these voices are very distressing. Just how distressing have they been?
MR A:	I have had enough.
DR T:	What do you mean?
MR A:	I can't stand it anymore.
DR T:	Can you tell me just what you mean?
MR A:	I am at the end of my tether. I can't go on like this. I have to kill myself.

Schizophrenia can also result in negative symptoms where patients are unable to experience feelings as acutely as before, and less able to think straight and marshall their thoughts. Such changes can be profoundly upsetting, especially to people who have creative abilities, such as artists. For example, a young artist who had an acute episode of schizophrenia developed blunting of affect. He complained that he was no longer able to feel the intense emotions which he required for his painting. This worried him because he felt it had impaired his ability to paint and the quality of his paintings had deteriorated.

When he received psychiatric treatment his acute symptoms (paranoid delusions and hallucinations) improved with medication. He also felt benefit from being on the ward and feeling he was in a supportive environment where the staff understood what was happening to him. After a few days he seemed to have improved considerably. The ward staff therefore considered that he was well enough to have two days' leave. During his leave he committed suicide. He went to his old school, of which he was very fond because he felt it had helped him to develop his interest in art. He climbed to the top of the school roof and jumped off. He left a note for his parents explaining that he could not contemplate life now that his affect was blunted and his painting was deteriorating. He did not believe that his affect would recover, although his acute symptoms had done so. He had not disclosed any of this to the treatment team. As discussed in Chapter 2, he thought the blunting of affect was inevitable and could not be corrected by treatment, and that there was therefore no point in mentioning it.

ALCOHOL AND SUBSTANCE ABUSE

Abuse of alcohol is associated with a much increased risk of suicide, especially when a person with an alcohol problem has suffered recent adverse life events such as a separation or job loss. After initial disinhibition, the alcohol acts as a depressant. If the patient is already clinically depressed, the risk of suicide can become extremely high. It is important, therefore, that you check for signs of dependence on alcohol, including increased or decreased tolerance, an overpowering need to drink (craving) regardless of the consequences, symptoms of withdrawal when stopping drinking (e.g. feeling shaky and tremulous) and memory lapses after even moderate drinking.

Unfortunately, when such patients present to Accident and Emergency or outpatient departments smelling of drink, it is tempting to send them away and insist that they sober up before any attempt is made to take a proper history and assess their mental state. Because of the risks involved, it is especially important to try to overcome your negative responses and determine whether such patients have felt depressed and thought of harming themselves. Similar caveats apply to those who admit they are suffering from drug abuse.

GENERALIZED ANXIETY AND PANIC DISORDERS

It is tempting for doctors to become habituated to high levels of distress when working in a hospital environment, and to take such distress for granted. It is then easy to underestimate the degree of torment that is caused by generalized anxiety disorder and spontaneous panic attacks. In panic disorder, the patient is suddenly overwhelmed by feelings of panic, and is terrified that they are dying. Yet intense anxiety and panic disorders are known to increase the risk of suicide because the patient believes this is the only way of escaping from the terror of dying that accompanies the attacks.

PERSONALITY DISORDER

The term 'personality disorder' is used to diagnose people who behave in such a consistently maladaptive way over time and across situations that they contribute to the negative events that occur in their lives. For example, they may experience repeated breakdowns in personal relationships because of their own behaviour, yet the breakdown of their relationships then provokes anxiety and depression, and problems with drink and drugs. If doctors think that a patient has a personality disorder, there is a high risk that they will devalue any symptoms of psychiatric illness such as depression, and that they will also minimize the risk of suicide. It is therefore important that you are careful when assessing such patients. Even though at a personal level you may dislike them and wish to cut the interview short, you should make every effort to assess whether concomitant mental illness is present and there is any risk of suicide.

GENERAL FACTORS THAT INCREASE SUICIDAL RISK

When you are assessing a patient and their history suggests that they are at risk of suicide, it is important to check whether any other key risk factors are present.

General factors that increase suicidal risk

- Social isolation
- Being recently separated or bereaved
- Loss of job
- Perceiving a lack of social support
- Chronic disabling or painful and life-threatening illness
- Being bereaved in early childhood
- Coming from a broken home
- Childlessness
- Being in a hostile dependent relationship
- Past history of suicide attempt(s)

ASSESSING THOSE DEEMED TO BE AT RISK

It is most important that you explore the patient's suicidal intent if there is evidence of them being at risk. The psychiatrist will take the referral seriously if you indicate that there is intent. It is mandatory that you ask 'Have you ever reached the point where you felt like ending your life?' Doctors are often reluctant to ask this question unless there is an obvious suicidal risk, because they fear the patient will be angered or upset by it. You should remember, therefore, that you are a professional who is performing an essential assessment task. Most patients who are feeling suicidal are relieved to be given an opportunity to talk about it.

Without explicit questioning, many suicidal patients will not disclose how they are feeling due to shame and embarrassment. If patients admit that they have thought about killing themselves, they must be asked 'Have you considered how you will do it?' 'Can you tell me just what you thought you might do?' They should then be encouraged to describe exactly what they have thought about doing. What matters when you are assessing their intent and plan is whether, from their viewpoint, the plan is likely to be successful. If the patient believes that taking only a few tablets would kill them, it is important to recognize that that is what is dictating their behaviour, even if the medical assessment suggests that such an overdose would not result in death.

It is also important to check the circumstances under which they plan to kill themselves, in order to determine whether there would be any likelihood that they would be found before they died, or if it is unlikely that they would be found. Thus if a patient claims he is going to kill himself by driving to a lonely place on the moors without having given any hint to anyone that he is clearly at high risk, you should be most concerned. Someone who plans to take some tablets knowing that their relative will be coming home in the next few minutes is at much less risk. If a patient has tried to commit suicide already, check how they felt about having failed ('How did you feel when you realized you were still alive?').

Some patients admit that although they have felt suicidal and had a plan, they have not been able to go through with it. It is important to establish what has stopped them. Common protective factors include religious beliefs that suicide is sinful or unacceptable, concern about how devastating it will be for their loved ones, fear of suffering pain and fear of failure.

You must then try to weigh the factors that suggest a high risk of suicide against those that appear to be protecting the patient. It can be difficult to determine the degree of risk when assessing depressed patients who are retarded but admit they feel suicidal. They may seem so slowed down and lacking in energy that they do not appear to have the ability to go through with a successful suicide attempt. There is a risk that once treatment of their depression has been started and they gain more energy they will be able to commit suicide before their mood has actually lifted. For this reason, knowing that a patient has been suicidal but is now on medication and seems to be improving should not prevent you from conducting a proper further risk assessment.

If patients are judged to be at high risk you have an immediate duty to protect them from harming themselves. They should be asked if they have any means of killing themselves on them, and invited to relinquish these articles. An immediate psychiatric opinion is required, but the patient should not be left alone while arrangements are being made for a psychiatric assessment. Someone must stay with them at all times so that they have no opportunity to kill themselves.

Some patients may be so depressed or deluded that they believe a disaster has either occurred already or will soon occur that will ruin the lives of their family as well as their own life. There is then a risk that they will kill their family before they kill themselves. For example, they may believe that some terrible misfortune (e.g. a bankruptcy) has befallen the family. They believe that there is now no future for them or the family, so they kill their family before killing themselves in order to protect them from the consequences. Therefore it is mandatory that you ask such patients 'How does that affect your view of your family's future? Is there any risk you want to protect them by taking them with you?'

On reading this you may feel that these are matters best left to a psychiatrist. However, unless the patient falls within a deliberate self-harm policy, they may not be automatically assessed by a specialist team. Similarly, if the patient is assessed in general practice it is most important that the degree of risk is properly established and an appropriate referral takes place. Unfortunately, newspapers continue to report inquests where a person has first killed several members of their family and then committed suicide because there was a failure to recognize the risk and act appropriately.

IMPACT OF EFFECTIVE COMMUNICATION

Most patients who feel suicidal, regardless of the underlying psychiatric disorder, personality problems or other factors involved, are ambivalent about it. While a major part of them wants to go through with a suicide attempt, there is usually a small part that wishes to be helped. Doctors who demonstrate a real willingness to understand how and why they are feeling suicidal are more likely to connect with the part of the patient that wants to go on living. It is most important that their reasons for suicide are not belittled but accepted, as that is how the patient sees things at the moment.

If the patient feels understood, this gives you some 'holding power', for they have come to respect your genuine attempts to understand what they are experiencing. This may then reduce the immediate risk of suicide because the patient begins to feel that something might be done to help them.

If the patient is at risk of suicide it is important that you are honest with them about what you think is going on. For example, you might say 'I am very concerned that you are at risk of going ahead and killing yourself because of how bad you are feeling. I think this is directly related to how depressed you have been. I think you have become depressed because of the stress of losing your wife. This has caused a biochemical change in your brain and your brain is now not producing certain chemicals that are crucial to maintain your normal mood. So you have been getting increasingly miserable and thinking more and more of suicide. I can understand that you feel, as a result of this, there is no point in going on living now that your wife has died and life feels so hopeless and empty. Suicide is also an attractive proposition because you believe it may result in you rejoining your wife. I need to explain though that we are likely to be able to treat this depression if you give us a chance to do so. Although you will still feel grief-stricken about losing your wife, you may be able to handle it more constructively. What I would like to do is ask a colleague of mine, a psychiatrist, to come and see you to decide what the best course of action would be'.

Patients usually feel relieved if they are given a rational explanation of why they are feeling so awful, and are also more likely to comply with your assessment and advice.

SUMMARY

It is mandatory to check with potentially suicidal patients whether they have specific and general features of risk. If there are any features of risk, it is important to ask the following key questions.

- Have you ever felt like ending your life?
- Have you ever considered a plan?
- What ways have you thought of?
- How close have you come to making an attempt?
- What exactly happened?
- Would you have any regrets if it didn't succeed?
- What has stopped you from making attempts so far?

If there is any suggestion of suicide, it is mandatory to obtain an urgent psychiatric opinion and to protect the patient from harming him- or herself in the mean time. It is also important to consider whether the patient has thought of harming anyone else.

chapter 10

HELPING THE BEREAVED

INTRODUCTION

The failure to grieve normally is associated with an increased risk of physical and psychiatric morbidity. Spouses of patients who died in general hospitals who failed to resolve their grief are at higher risk of developing common physical illnesses such as heart disease, cancer and problems with blood pressure (Prigerson *et al.*, 1997). The psychiatric morbidity that results includes generalized anxiety disorder, depressive illness, alcoholism, hypochondriasis and agoraphobia (Parkes and Markus, 1998). When bereaved people develop depression and/or alcoholism, there is a greatly increased risk that they will commit suicide. This risk of suicide continues for up to 8 years after the bereavement, and is particularly likely to occur at the time of important events such as birthdays or wedding anniversaries.

Failure to grieve has longer-term consequences in that it makes individuals more vulnerable to subsequent losses. For example, women who lost their mother in childhood are at much greater risk of developing mental illness than those who did not experience such loss, when in adulthood they experience stressful life events which threaten some form of loss, such as a loss of job or health. The loss of a parent in early life has also been found to have a negative effect on the ability of individuals to form and maintain relationships in adulthood. Those who have experienced sudden loss in childhood may, when they attempt new relationships, become fearful that such abandonment by death may occur again. This may result in them either avoiding relationships altogether or becoming too dependent and clingy.

Unfortunately, the way in which death is managed within hospitals and general practice may hinder the resolution of grief. Even when patterns of abnormal grief develop they often go unrecognized until there is major physical or psychiatric morbidity. Yet doctors who are confronted by the death of their patients are in a strong position to facilitate the process of grieving.

OBJECTIVES

The objectives of this chapter are to:

- discuss strategies that will allow you to facilitate grieving in the context of:
    perinatal death;
    sudden unexpected death;

contd

patients who are brought in dead;

death within the home;

- discuss how to deal with particularly challenging situations:

  requesting a post-mortem;

  requesting organ donation;

- describe normal grief;

- describe patterns of abnormal/traumatic grief:

  absent grief;

  delayed grief;

  oscillating grief;

  chronic grief;

  exploding grief;

- describe markers of abnormal grief;

- discuss key risk factors;

- describe how to assist the bereaved, distinguish between normal and abnormal grief and decide whether or not psychological intervention is needed.

FACILITATING GRIEVING

PERINATAL DEATH

The loss of a child prematurely or at the time of birth is especially traumatic to parents. It runs counter to all of their positive expectations and comes as a shock and bitter disappointment. It is often sudden and unexpected, and there is therefore a high risk that the parents, especially the mother, will try to block out the painful reality, particularly if the mother is suffering from the after-effects of anaesthetics or other drugs. For this reason, you should use strategies that will help her to confront reality.

Confront reality and be honest about the circumstances

You should make every effort, however painful it may be, to help the mother to confront reality by being honest about the fact that the child has died, explaining explicitly the circumstances of the death and checking that she has absorbed this information accurately.

Encourage holding of the baby and saying goodbye

If possible, the mother should be encouraged to hold the baby and relate to it. Provided that she can tolerate this, she must also be encouraged to say goodbye to the baby before it is taken from her.

Negotiate about photographs

You should then negotiate to see if she wishes to be left with a photograph of the baby to act as a reminder of her loss. A similar discussion should take place with the father.

When doctors delay telling parents that their baby is dead or try to cover up the circumstances surrounding the death, this increases the risk that the parents will deny that death has occurred or fantasize in an unhelpful way about how the child came to die. They may believe that the hospital or the doctors involved were responsible for the death.

GROSS PHYSICAL ABNORMALITY

When a child has been born prematurely or died at full term because of a gross physical abnormality, you should warn the parents about this and check whether they still wish to see the child and have a photograph taken. Most parents are still comforted by having a photograph, regardless of the abnormality involved. As with perinatal death, if there is no negotiation and the child is withheld from them, they may feel bitter because they believe that the hospital caused the death. Confronting the parents with the loss of their baby, whether accompanied by gross physical abnormality or not, is an extremely painful task. Advice on how you might cope with your feelings in this situation is given in Chapter 11. Remember that facilitating grief using these strategies has a profoundly beneficial effect on the parents in the longer term, even though it causes enormous upset initially. Parents highly respect doctors who are willing to bear the brunt of telling such bad news and explaining the circumstances.

HANDLING THE AFTERMATH

When telling parents about the death of their child, it is important to negotiate whether they wish to be left alone to grieve together or would prefer to talk to you about how they are feeling. You should encourage them to grieve by saying it is normal for people to be extremely upset in these circumstances, and they must feel free to express and talk about their feelings if they wish to do so. It is most important that you add that you will be willing to stay with them while they do this, and are empathic ('It must be a desperate disappointment given how much you were looking forward to this baby'). You should avoid any attempt to make apparently reassuring statements, such as 'I know you are upset but I am sure you will be able to have another one', for nothing you can say will soften the reality of their facing the loss of their child. Instead, you should ask them directly if they have any questions about the nature and circumstances of the baby's death, if they have any other concerns and whether they feel they need any help.

Summary of steps to take when dealing with the aftermath of child death

- Negotiate if they wish to talk
- Legitimize their distress
- Be empathic
- Screen for any questions and concerns
- Check how they are feeling
- Check whether they feel that they need any practical or psychological help

SUDDEN UNEXPECTED DEATH

Unfortunately, some patients die without there being warning that they are going to do so. Doctors or nurses in this situation may have advised relatives that it was safe for them to take time out from being with the patient and go home and get some much-needed rest. If the patient then dies unexpectedly, the relatives may feel guilty that they did not stay despite the doctors' and nurses' advice. Alternatively, they may believe that the death occurred because inadequate care was given and there was negligence.

You must therefore be prepared to meet with the relatives as soon as possible after the death, rather than fob them off and leave non-medical people to explain the circumstances of the death. You should confirm that death has occurred ('I am sorry to have to tell you that she died 90 minutes ago') and confirm that it was unexpected ('As you know, we were not expecting her to die so soon'). It is also helpful to apologize ('I am sorry we were not able to warn you so you could be here at the time'). Most relatives will accept this and will then want to know the exact circumstances of the death. However, others will not want to know the details. Therefore it is important that you negotiate ('Do you want to know exactly what happened?') and then explain the precise circumstances. You should also give them a chance to ask any questions ('Have you any questions?') rather than volunteer information ('She died quietly', 'She wasn't suffering unduly' or 'We don't think she suffered') before they have voiced their concerns.

Summary of action to take in the event of sudden unexpected death

- Meet with the relatives soon
- Confirm that death has occurred
- Explain that it was unexpected
- Apologize that they could not be forewarned
- Check whether they want details
- Ask if they have any questions
- Do not volunteer information that is not asked for

When relatives are angry it is important to respond to their anger as discussed in Chapter 7. They may also feel guilty that they were not present at the time of death or able to say goodbye. You should legitimize this and say 'Given the circumstances, there is no way in which you could have been there, as we advised you it was all right to go home and rest'.

VIEWING THE BODY

After confirming that death has occurred and inviting an initial discussion, you must check whether the relatives wish to view the patient's body. Some relatives prefer to leave witnessing and saying goodbye until the body is in the Chapel of Rest, when the undertaker has been able to prepare the body appropriately. Others may wish to see the body immediately. If the manner of death was unpleasant, it is important to warn relatives and to negotiate whether they still wish to see the patient's body. If they decide to view the body in hospital, it is important to inform them that they are welcome to talk to you again afterwards about what has happened.

ENCOURAGING THE EXPRESSION OF FEELINGS

At such a traumatic time when relatives are confronting unexpected death they are likely to become tearful. You should acknowledge this and give them permission to cry openly by saying 'I can see you are upset. It is important that you try to let your feelings out now if you can, and talk about exactly what is distressing you'. As they talk, you should explore the reasons for their distress and summarize their concerns. This maximizes the likelihood that they will grieve normally.

You should also check whether they want help with practical matters such as the death certificate and personal property, and explain that if they have any further questions they should get back in touch with you to discuss them. In summary, you should encourage the expression of feelings by adopting the following approach.

Summary of action to take to encourage expression of feelings

- Acknowledge the relatives' distress
- Encourage expression of feelings
- Explore the main reasons for distress
- Check whether the relatives have any other concerns
- Summarize their concerns
- Check whether they need help
- Offer further contact

Remember that most individuals who are bereaved in this way are psychologically robust and capable of working through their grief. If you give them accurate and true information and allow them to respond accordingly, they are far more likely to cope effectively. However well you deal with this situation, though, some relatives will remain very distressed. It is important to check if there is someone you can call to collect them, take them home and support them for the next 48 or 72 hours.

PATIENTS WHO ARE BROUGHT IN DEAD

Major problems arise when relatives come into hospital believing that the patient is still alive. They may think that resuscitation has worked and they will soon be reunited with their loved ones. Often they will have been the subject of false reassurance given by doctors, ambulance personnel or policemen who may have said, for example, 'Oh, I know he is very ill but I am sure we can bring him round'.

It is important that you negotiate with the relatives if they wish to be present during efforts at resuscitation. Some relatives will wish to be there in order to be with their loved one and ensure that everything possible has been done. Others may not want to be involved and prefer to wait outside, where they can be contacted once the result is known.

If resuscitation is not possible, it is important that there is no pretence that the patient is still alive. Instead, you must give the relatives a realistic account of what has happened. For example, 'I am afraid his heart stopped twice on the way here in the ambulance. He was already dead when he arrived'. If the resuscitation is ongoing, it is important that the relatives are given a realistic account ('We are doing our best to revive him, but it doesn't look hopeful'). This prepares the relatives for the worst, and it is then more likely they will assimilate the death, begin to come to terms with it and grieve appropriately than if they have been fobbed off by comforting but untruthful statements. If they are misled and then told that death has occurred, they may believe that the patient died because of mistakes that were made while he or she was in hospital.

DEATH IN THE HOME

General practitioners may find it especially difficult to deal with deaths in the home, for they are likely to have known the patients and their families for some time. They may therefore experience the loss as personal and find it very painful to deal with. They may feel as perplexed as the family when the death is unexpected, and may also feel angry if a young adult or child has died. If they were the doctor on call and had no prior contact with the family, they may feel at a distinct disadvantage and be tempted to deal with the relatives' distress by advising sedation and leaving the house as soon as possible. However, the use of anxiolytic drugs such as benzodiazepines is inadvisable, as they can block the expression of grief. If sedation has to be given, low doses of major tranquillizers (e.g. thioridizine, 25–50 mg t.i.d.) are more advisable.

Even in the home, doctors should be willing to acknowledge the pain and distress involved, be empathic and check whether the relatives wish and can bear to talk about what has happened and express their feelings. They should identify their main concerns and establish what help, if any, they need. If the cause of death is uncertain, the doctor may have to explain that a post-mortem examination will be needed.

REQUESTING A POST-MORTEM

The need for a post-mortem should not be discussed until you have first established the relatives' views about what has happened and their feelings. Otherwise, they are likely to perceive you as uncaring and insensitive, and may become very angry. Once their views and feelings have been established, you should break the bad news in an empathic way.

DR J: As we discussed, I have no idea why Anne has died. It was totally out of the blue. Unfortunately, that means there will have to be a post-mortem to try and find out why she died. I guess that's the last thing you wanted to hear just now.

MRS P: I can't bear the thought of her being cut up. Is there no other way? It's bad enough losing her without that.

DR J: I wish there was another way but I am afraid there isn't. It's legally necessary. However, it might actually be of help if you knew why she had died.

MRS P: I suppose so, otherwise I will keep torturing myself that there was something I should have noticed, could have done.

In this example, the doctor did not try to soften the bad news about the post-mortem by volunteering statements such as 'She's dead, she won't feel anything' or 'the pathologist will be very gentle'. Once you have explained that the post-mortem is necessary, it is important to check with the relatives whether they have concerns about the post-mortem, and to explore these.

REQUESTING ORGAN DONATION

Young doctors working in hospital can find themselves in a difficult situation if a patient is judged to be 'brain-dead' but their other main organs are fully functioning. They may be under pressure to ask for organ donation. This is a potential minefield emotionally, especially if the dead person did not carry a donor card or make their wishes explicit. It is important that you make a real effort to understand the consequences of the death for the relatives, and try to 'get alongside them' in their predicament concerning the implications of losing the patient. They will then be much more willing to consider the possibility that one way of salvaging something positive from the situation might be to consider organ donation.

You should begin by focusing on the issue directly ('Have you ever thought about the issue of people donating their organs for transplantation to others?'). If they have, the doctor can ask 'What are your feelings about it?' If this reveals strong emotional resistance, there is no point moving into logical persuasion mode ('If you agree to her organs being donated, her death will not have been in vain'). Instead, you should respect and acknowledge their resistance ('I can see you find the idea distasteful, so I won't pursue it any further').

In contrast, if the relatives are sympathetic to the idea you should explore their reasons ('What exactly makes you support the idea of organ donation?') and then determine whether their reasons are appropriate. If their ideas are unrealistic you should explain the likely real benefits and risks.

The use of these communication strategies in the contexts discussed will do much to help you prevent abnormal grief patterns. However, it is still important that you are able to distinguish between abnormal and normal grief for the reasons discussed previously.

NORMAL GRIEF

If the grief process is to begin, the bereaved person has to acknowledge both intellectually and emotionally that death has occurred. The phases of normal grief are discussed in turn.

Emotional acceptance of loss

If members of the family were present at the death, the period of numbness and shock should last only a few days at most. The onset of grief should then be obvious through their descriptions of experiencing intrusive waves of strong feelings like a sense of loss, sadness, despair, anger or guilt. When people feel overwhelmed by these feelings they may complain of feeling 'confused' and find it difficult to say exactly what they are feeling. Between these periods of intrusive waves of grief the person who has been recently bereaved will feel either calm or apathetic.

Burial or cremation is a public signal that death has occurred, and it allows family and friends to mourn openly. The waves of grief then escalate in their frequency, duration and intensity until they reach a natural plateau. At this point individuals are grieving maximally but do not feel in danger of 'going mad' or being overwhelmed by their grief. A key feature of normal grief is the ability of individuals to allow their grief to emerge, and their preparedness to express it whether in public or in private.

Perceptual phenomena

During the period immediately after bereavement, the relatives often experience a strong sense of the presence of the dead person. This can be comforting, but then it also reminds them that the dead person is no longer there, and thus can provoke further waves of grief. They may experience illusions in which they see other people who they think look like the dead person, but once they are close to them they realize it is an illusion. They might experience hallucinations in which they see or hear the dead person, but they soon realize that this was a trick of their imagination. It is common for the bereaved to feel restless. They may find themselves pacing within the house and going from room to room or visiting places where they might have found the dead person when he or she was alive. These behaviours represent primitive searching and are a biological attempt to re-establish a bond with the dead person.

Mental distress

Shortly after bereavement, the relatives may complain of feeling anxious, depressed and even suicidal. In contrast to the symptoms associated with generalized anxiety disorder, major depressive illness and suicidal ideation, these feelings are usually fleeting and sporadic. Occasional feelings of irritability, impaired concentration and poor memory are also common.

Physical symptoms

Recently bereaved people also complain of various physical symptoms, notably palpitations, chest pain, dizziness, feeling drained and various aches and pains.

Such symptoms should be taken seriously in the first instance, to eliminate the risk that they may have developed serious physical illness such as heart disease. However, it is also important that you check whether these symptoms represent identification reactions, where the symptoms they have been experiencing mimic exactly those that were experienced by the dead person during the last few weeks of life.

RESOLUTION

In most individuals the period of maximum grief lasts for 8 to 12 weeks. They then notice that the waves of grief are becoming less frequent, less intense, and shorter in duration. This pattern of normal grief can be represented diagrammatically (Figure 10.1). Once such a slope has been developed, it can take a considerable time for a person to stop experiencing these phenomena. Most people will return to normal after the first anniversary and within 2 or 3 years after the death.

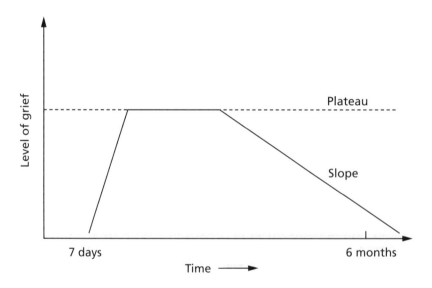

Figure 10.1 Normal grief

MARKERS OF NORMAL GRIEF

The following markers indicate that a relative is grieving normally. It is important, therefore, to ask about these directly.

- Acknowledgement that they have accepted that the person is dead at an emotional level
- Confronting the reality of loss by attending the funeral or cremation
- Able to let go of key belongings
- Able to connect with happy memories

contd

- Visiting the cemetery or crematorium at reasonable intervals
- Able to look at photographs and feel both comforted and upset
- A decrease in the frequency and intensity of their waves of grief.
- A decrease in their preoccupation with thoughts of the dead person
- Frequent illusions, hallucinations or searching behaviour

When such normal grief is occurring, relatives do not need intervention, although they will benefit from feeling that you have tried to understand what they are going through.

ABNORMAL/TRAUMATIC GRIEF

It is most important that you can recognize when these patterns are evident.

Patterns of abnormal grief

- Absent grief
- Delayed grief
- Oscillating grief
- Chronic grief
- Exploding grief

ABSENT GRIEF

In absent grief there is no evidence that the person is grieving, despite their experiencing the reality of death. This signifies that the reality is too painful for them. Thus if you ask them whether they have experienced any grief following the bereavement, they will say they have not. They may also volunteer that they have not been able to accept that the person has died, and believe that he or she will return home at any moment.

For example, a man whose wife died of breast cancer could not accept that she was dead. Although he knew logically that she had died, he could not face the reality emotionally. When he attended the funeral he felt that he was in a dream and that it was happening to someone else. After his wife died he kept the house immaculately tidy on the grounds that she would return home soon and he owed it to her because she was so house-proud. He left the bedroom exactly as it was before she died, and had not removed any photographs or belongings. He did not believe there was any point in visiting the cemetery because in his view she was not there (Figure 10.2).

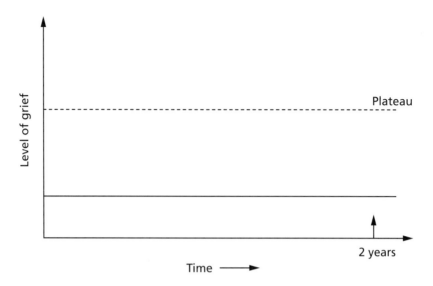

Figure 10.2 Absent grief

DELAYED GRIEF

In delayed grief the bereaved person makes a conscious effort to avoid grieving. They may often explain this on the basis that they have to carry on normally because of the needs of their family or business. They distract themselves deliberately so that they do not have time to grieve. Eventually, their grief is triggered by a strong reminder that the person has died – this may be the time of an anniversary or some other key event (Figure 10.3).

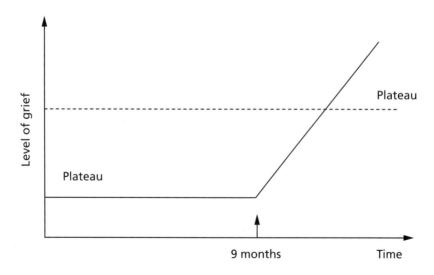

Figure 10.3 Delayed grief

OSCILLATING GRIEF

This tends to be associated with deaths which have been violent and unpleasant (e.g. through road traffic accidents, assault or murder). The bereaved person is then confronted with extremely unpleasant images that are too painful to face. They try to allow these to emerge and begin to grieve, but then find that the pain is so great that they have no alternative but to suppress the images. Mental suppression of images and memories requires a large amount of mental energy. Within only a few months the bereaved person will have used up all the psychological energy available. Their grief then emerges, begins to overwhelm them, and can lead to major anxiety, depression and risk of suicide (Figure 10.4)

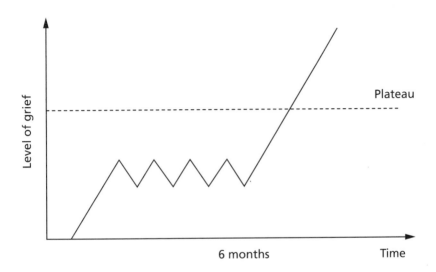

Figure 10.4 Oscillating grief

CHRONIC GRIEF

During the first few weeks after death the grief appears to be progressing normally. However, once it has hit the natural plateau it remains there, and there is no evidence of any slope developing. Such individuals are reluctant to let go of belongings, and they avoid visiting the cemetery or crematorium and looking at photographs. They are trying to hang on to the dead person because of a deep underlying fear of emptiness, loneliness and desolation (Figure 10.5).

EXPLODING GRIEF

Here, grief develops as normal but then accelerates beyond the normal plateau. The bereaved person feels overwhelmed by their feelings and expresses fears that they are 'going crazy'. Such individuals require urgent help if they are not to be seriously affected by major depression and anxiety (Figure 10.6).

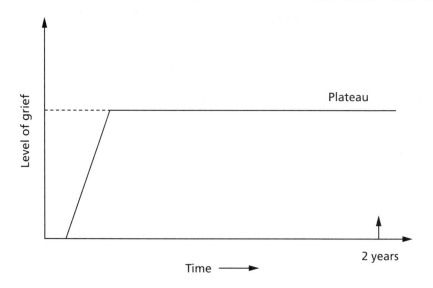

Figure 10.5 Chronic grief

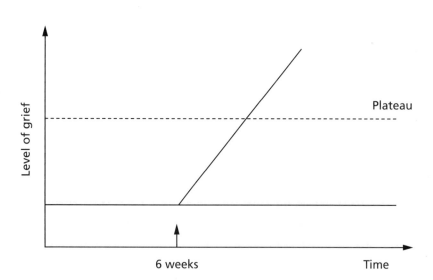

Figure 10.6 Exploding grief

MARKERS OF ABNORMAL GRIEF

The following markers need to be enquired about as part of an assessment if you suspect that grief may not be proceeding normally.

- Avoidance of seeing the body, or refusal to be parted from it
- Avoidance of burial or cremation
- Avoidance of or excessive visits to the cemetery/crematorium
- Absence or excess presence of photographs in the house
- Evidence of maintaining a shrine to the dead person
- Refusal to let go of the dead person's belongings
- Inability to connect with positive memories
- No lessening in the frequency and intensity of grief, preoccupations, searching, illusions or hallucinations

RISK FACTORS FOR ABNORMAL GRIEF

The following risk factors have been established which render individuals susceptible to developing abnormal patterns of grief.

- Mutually dependent, over-dependent, ambivalent or skewed relationships
- Sudden, unexpected, stormy or violent death
- Perceiving that the death was preventable by self or others
- Death leading to unfinished, thwarted wishes and ambitions
- Perceived lack of support
- Experiencing other life crises at the same time
- Competing responsibilities

NATURE OF RELATIONSHIP

Individuals with a strong but mutual dependence are especially at risk, as they will not have needed or utilized other friends for support or comfort at times of crisis. Thus the loss of a partner leaves a huge hole in their lives. Individuals who were over-dependent on the other person are left abandoned when that individual dies. They may have been protected from having to make simple decisions such as whether and when to pay bills, and are therefore ill prepared for sudden and unwanted autonomy. Those who had strongly ambivalent relationships, where they both loved and hated the other person, can feel especially guilty at their death, and this may block their grief.

Some individuals develop a skewed relationship. For example, a woman may have had a reasonable relationship with her husband but sensed that there was something missing. She may then bear a child who develops a loving, sparkling personality, and to whom the mother increasingly turns for emotional satisfaction. The child becomes ill, and during the child's illness she spends increasing amounts of time being involved in her treatment and care. The mother may spend many days in hospital before the child dies. At this time she feels extremely bitter and angry that the child who mattered most has been taken from her, yet she is also physically and emotionally exhausted because of the time she has spent caring for the child. She has become disfranchised from her partner and her other children, who all feel neglected, so she is unlikely to get the necessary emotional support at the time of the death. For all these reasons she will be vulnerable to major depression.

CIRCUMSTANCES OF DEATH

Death which is sudden and unexpected and takes a violent form is especially difficult to come to terms with, especially if the grieving person cannot view the body.

It is important, therefore, that you try to encourage relatives to take time out from looking after an ill person or visiting hospital so frequently when the images they may be left with are harsh, and they may use up all of their available energy.

PREVENTABILITY

It is difficult for relatives to grieve if they believe that the death could have been prevented if they or other people had behaved differently. For example, a woman was married to a man who complained frequently about various physical symptoms, including chest pain. He had been seen repeatedly by doctors who said there was nothing wrong with him. One night he complained yet again that he was experiencing chest pain. He said he was going upstairs to lie down. She paid no heed to this because it seemed no different to his usual behaviour. After an hour she began to worry about him and went upstairs to find him dead. She could not stop thinking about the fact that if only she had checked sooner she might have found that he was ill and could have summoned medical help which might have prevented his death.

TIME OF DEATH

The ability to resolve grief is proportional to the amount of unfinished emotional and practical business that is left. When important ambitions have been thwarted (e.g. when a couple experiences a still birth) it is especially important to look for signs of abnormal grief patterns afterwards.

PERCEIVED LACK OF SUPPORT

A major factor in promoting normal grief is the feeling that others around the bereaved person understand what they have gone through and are prepared to support them. Many people remember for the rest of their lives how helpful a doctor was at the time of a sudden unpleasant death, in that the doctor was willing to try to understand their predicament, concerns and feelings and be supportive, and avoided giving them false and unhelpful reassurance.

OTHER LIFE CRISES

Having to contend with other major problems at the time of bereavement can inhibit the ability of the recently bereaved to deal with the death.

COMPETING RESPONSIBILITIES

People who have to keep going for the sake of their family, business or job may not take enough time out to grieve. However, it is likely that they may use these responsibilities as alibis to avoid facing the painful reality of what has happened.

ASSESSMENT

When taking a history of a patient's presenting complaints, you may find that the patient has had a recent bereavement. It is important that you check whether they are prepared to talk about it ('It sounds like the death of your mother 2 years ago may still be a problem for you. I realize that talking about it could be upsetting for you. Can I check that you are prepared to do so?'). It is important that you say 'If at any stage it gets too painful for you, you must tell me and I'll stop'. This negotiation should be made genuinely, so that if the patient indicates it is too painful you will heed this and not pursue it any further.

You should invite the patient to talk about the exact circumstances of the bereavement. This will make it more likely that they can connect with the key events and recall the actual feelings.

Dr S: When exactly did your mother die?
Mrs H: 1995.
Dr S: Can you remember the exact day?
Mrs H: August 22nd.
Dr S: What time of day?
Mrs H: Seven o'clock in the evening.

Dr S next asks 'Can you bear to tell me exactly what happened?' He also asks specific questions, including whether she was present at the time of death, how the death occurred, and how she felt about the circumstances ('She looked at peace' or 'She died in terrible pain'). If she was not present it is important for him to ask 'Why not?', and he checks whether the relative saw the body at any stage, checks how she reacted to seeing the body and asks whether she had any regrets about not being there at the time of death. It is also important for the doctor to check whether the patient was buried or cremated, and if the relative was able to go to the ceremony, how she reacted ('It was as though it was in a film and happening to someone else' or 'It was heartbreaking. I was losing my best friend'). It is crucial to map out the frequency, intensity, nature and duration of any waves of grief over the next few weeks in order to allow the doctor to assess any changes that occur subsequently. It is also important to establish whether the patient was able to express their feelings openly or hid or suppressed them.

Similarly, the doctor should establish how preoccupied the patient was during the first few weeks of bereavement with thoughts of the dead person both during the day and at night-time, and whether the patient has suffered from such preoccupation in the form of nightmares. The extent of any searching, sense of presence, illusions and hallucinations should also be determined. It is then possible for the doctor to compare how the patient is coping now with how they were coping during the first few weeks after the death. This will indicate if a slope has developed and the phenomena of grief are lessening in frequency and intensity. If there is no evident slope and the abnormal pattern of grief is present, the doctor must check whether the patient has been able to let go of the dead person's belongings, is able to look at photographs of them, has been able to visit the cemetery or crematorium, and is able to connect with positive memories.

When the pattern of grief appears abnormal (traumatic), the doctor should check whether any possible risk factors have been present. These should include the nature of the patient's relationship with the dead person, why the patient feels it has been difficult to come to terms with their death, whether there were other life crises at the time of the death, whether the death could have been prevented in any way, whether key ambitions and plans have been thwarted, whether the patient feels that sufficient emotional and practical support has been forthcoming, and whether any other factors were present that may have blocked the grief.

If the pattern is one of attenuated slope or chronic grief, taking a history as described above may unlock the grief in a productive way. The patient will then cry as the experience of bereavement is described, and this may lead to proper resolution of the grief. If this fails or the other patterns of abnormal grief are evident, you should consider referral to a bereavement counsellor, clinical psychologist or psychiatrist to accelerate the bereavement process and reduce the risk of major physical and psychiatric morbidity.

SUMMARY

You are in a key position to facilitate grieving in those who are suddenly bereaved by acknowledging honestly the reality of loss and giving the relatives an opportunity to talk about this, express their feelings and ask any relevant questions. You must be alert to the presence of abnormal patterns of grief in bereaved patients, be able to distinguish between abnormal and normal patterns, and encourage patients to seek help where appropriate.

REFERENCES

Parkes, C.M. and Markus, A. (eds) 1998: *Coping with loss*. London: BMJ Books.

Prigerson, H.G., Bierhals, A.J., Stanislav, M.P.H. *et al.* 1997: Traumatic grief as a risk factor for mental and physical morbidity. *American Journal of Psychiatry* 154, 616–22.

HOW TO COMMUNICATE EFFECTIVELY AND SURVIVE EMOTIONALLY

INTRODUCTION

As a profession, doctors are known to be at increased risk of developing mental illnesses such as generalized anxiety disorder, major depressive illness, alcohol and/or drug abuse. The development of these disorders is often preceded by a period of 'burnout'. This consists of the following three elements:

- depersonalization;
- emotional exhaustion;
- low levels of personal achievement.

Depersonalization is said to have occurred when doctors begin to relate to patients and relatives in a detached and unfeeling way. Emotional exhaustion refers to the situation where doctors have become worn out emotionally and have no reserves left. They become increasingly tired and so find their work demands much more effort. Low personal achievement indicates they feel that they are achieving much less in their job, are deriving little if any job satisfaction, and are questioning whether there is much value in what they are doing.

OBJECTIVES

The objectives of this final chapter are to review

- the prevalence of burnout in senior doctors, and the factors associated with it;
- the prevalence of stress in medical students, and the factors associated with it;
- strategies to minimize burnout and enhance personal survival;
- how to develop self-awareness;
- how to improve communication skills.

BURNOUT IN SENIOR DOCTORS

Ramirez and her colleagues studied burnout in 882 senior cancer doctors, including gastroenterologists, surgeons, radiologists and oncologists (Ramirez *et al.*, 1995). They found that between 25% and 33% had high levels of emotional exhaustion, 20% to 25% had high levels of depersonalization while 33% to 50% reported low levels of personal achievement. About 25% of the sample obtained scores on the General Health Questionnaire which suggested that they were possible 'cases' of mood disorder. There was a strong relationship between high burnout scores and high scores on the General Health Questionnaire.

Factors that appeared to contribute to doctors developing burnout included their feeling dissatisfied with their ability to relate to patients, relatives and staff. A major factor concerned their feeling that they had been trained inadequately in key communication skills and tasks. They also had concerns about their professional status and felt that they lacked intellectual stimulation. They worried that they were being less effective with their patients than they should be because they lacked key communication skills. They felt frustrated about this, and guilty and worried about the adverse consequences it might have for patients and their families.

Doctors with high burnout scores were concerned that when they confronted patients' suffering but were unable to cure their disease, this provoked strong feelings of powerlessness and led them to believe that both they as individuals and medicine as a profession had failed patients and their families. They felt that they had no constructive way of dealing with their own anger, frustration and guilt, and they tended to suppress their feelings and did not discuss them with anyone. Other important factors included feeling overwhelmed by their workload, and worrying about the negative impact that this was having on their life at home and particularly their personal relationships. They considered that they were given insufficient resources to deal with their workload, and they felt poorly managed.

STRESS IN MEDICAL STUDENTS

Undue stress is apparent even in medical students. It was found that 31% of a sample of medical students studied by Firth-Cousins (1989) showed evidence of mood disturbance. This was defined as a score of 4 or more on a 12-item General Health Questionnaire. The 'probable caseness rate' was three times that found in a comparison group of young unemployed people. There was also evidence of an increase in students' drinking habits during their clinical years.

The nature of the stressors that they experienced was similar to those reported by the cancer specialists. Around 20% of the events most commonly reported as stressful involved talking to patients, particularly psychiatric patients. In total, 12% of students were concerned about the adverse effects of their studies on their private lives, particularly their personal relationships and finances, and 12% reported that they experienced stress when presenting cases, usually feeling humiliated by their consultants, while 10% found it difficult to deal with the suffering and death that they encountered. The two factors that made them most upset and led to them feeling frustrated, tense and powerless were their relationships with their consultants, and feeling that medicine had failed their patients.

When asked to complete a check-list of events that they found particularly stressful, 34% cited their relationship with their consultants, 31% cited the effect on their personal lives and 24% cited talking to terminally ill patients. They found it especially difficult to deal with suffering and death, particularly talking to recently bereaved relatives when the patient had died suddenly and unexpectedly. They did not feel overworked as medical students, but said that the most unsatisfactory aspect of their role was feeling useless and not contributing directly to patient care. Although they most enjoyed talking to patients, they felt that they were given insufficient opportunity to do so. They also lacked confidence in their ability to talk to patients because they believed they lacked training in key communication skills.

A recent study of doctors in the workplace suggested that the following practical factors contribute to this stress.

- Noisy on-call rooms which interfere with sleep
- No provision of hot food at night
- No control over their workload
- Inadequate career counselling
- Poor channels of communication
- Limited opportunities for study and research
- Pressure on beds
- Cancellation of routine work
- Business ethos within hospitals and general practice
- Shortages of nursing staff
- Feeling underpaid and undervalued

NEED FOR PERSONAL REFLECTION

Given the nature, magnitude and prevalence of these stressors, it is important for medical students and young doctors to reflect on how their studies and work are affecting their lives. Novack *et al.* (1998) have suggested that this should be done systematically so that medical students and doctors become aware if they are suffering from major stressors, can identify their source, and can find ways of modifying the stressors before they cause burnout and lead to psychiatric problems. Novack and colleagues believe that personal reflection must cover specific aspects of doctors' attitudes and behaviour if they are to develop appropriate self-awareness and take appropriate action. These aspects are listed below.

- Doctors' beliefs and attitudes
    Core beliefs
    Influence of family of origin
    Gender issues
    Socio-cultural influences

- Emotional responses to patient care
  - Caring for patients
  - Anger and conflict
- Challenging clinical situations
  - Difficult patients
  - Dying patients
  - Medical mistakes
- Doctors' self-care

DOCTORS' BELIEFS AND ATTITUDES

Core beliefs

Medical students and doctors ought to know their core beliefs and attitudes about life in general, themselves as individuals, the role of medicine and their attitude to others. You should ask yourself the following questions: 'How available do I need to be to my patients?', 'What are the scope and limits of my responsibility to them?' and 'Should I treat patients with psychosocial and mental health problems?'

Doctors appear to be more at risk of burnout if they believe that any limitations of their professional knowledge represent a personal failing, that they should bear the responsibility for patient care alone, that denial of their own personal needs is desirable or that their own uncertainties and emotions must be kept private.

Influence of family of origin

Medical students and young doctors need to reflect on the impact of their family of origin on their attitudes and behaviour with regard to their work. The areas covered should include consideration of intimacy with others, handling of anger, and how they deal with conflict. Beliefs about the nature, benefits and disadvantages of caring, the roles of caregivers, the balance of giving vs. receiving help, communicating about illness and responding to stress can all be strongly influenced by their experiences within their own families.

Medical students and doctors may identify consciously or unconsciously with patients who present with similar problems to those they experienced in members of their own families. This can provoke strong fears that they may harm patients, that they are personally inadequate, and that they may lose control emotionally, or avoid or become over-involved with the patient. Therefore some useful questions you should consider include 'What roles did I have in my family?', 'Am I replicating these in my work?', 'What lessons did I learn about relationships, caregiving and responding to ill people?', 'What kinds of people remind me of family members?' and 'How do I react?'.

Gender issues

More male than female doctors are likely to believe that female patients have a psychosomatic or functional basis to their illness and are more demanding, despite a lack of objective evidence to justify this view. Male doctors tend to patronize female patients, so it is important to address the following questions.

- What messages did I receive about gender roles from my family in particular, and society in general?
- Have my attitudes about gender led to problems in communication with the opposite sex?
- Do I respond differently to male and female patients?
- Do they respond differently to me?
- Do I respond differently to feedback from male and female colleagues?

Socio-cultural influences

Many medical students and doctors in the UK come from overseas and from different cultures. Similarly, a growing number of patients and relatives are from ethnic minorities. The influence of social class also needs to be considered. For example, medical students and doctors may have strong prejudices about patients presenting with 'illness behaviour', suffering from obesity or advocating particular sexual behaviours, and about the elderly and patients from other cultures. You must therefore ask the following questions.

- To what culture do I belong?
- With what culture do I identify?
- What values do I particularly like or dislike?
- When interacting with people from other cultures, what factors help me to feel comfortable rather than uncomfortable?
- How has my medical training affected my attitudes?
- What is the culture within my institution or practice?

EMOTIONAL RESPONSES TO PATIENT CARE

Caring for patients

Caring for and being concerned about patients is essential if medical practice is to be effective. However, it is only beneficial if it is kept within clear and mutually understood boundaries, otherwise, there may be a danger of sending unintentional messages which result in the doctor or patient becoming too involved emotionally. This is especially true if the patient and doctor know each other socially. In any doctor–patient relationship there is the potential for powerful feelings of attraction to develop given the intimacy of this relationship. The doctor may defend him- or herself against this by becoming too detached, or he or she may become too involved, even to the point of having a sexual relationship with the patient. It is crucial that you reflect on your emotional reactions to your patients and the possible sources of these reactions.

Anger and conflict

If anger and conflict are not handled properly they can prove destructive to a relationship. You therefore need to develop awareness about what triggers anger in you and how you react to conflict in your relationships with patients and colleagues. If you find it difficult to manage conflict, you will need to develop strategies that allow you to do so.

Useful questions include the following.

- What types of patients make me angry?
- What work situations make me angry, and why?
- How do I usually respond to anger (including both my own anger and that of others)?
- Do I tend to over-react, placate, blame, suppress or become super-reasonable?
- What are my underlying feelings when I become angry?
- Do they include feeling rejected, humiliated, unworthy and devalued?
- Where did I learn these responses?
- Do I have any alternatives at my disposal?

CHALLENGING CLINICAL SITUATIONS

Difficult patients

Medical students and doctors inevitably encounter some patients whom they view as 'difficult'. Such patients have been described as 'heart-sink' patients. They generally have symptoms that cannot be understood and which do not improve, even when the correct treatments appear to have been given. These patients often have major stresses in their lives and a past history of psychiatric illness. They have more functional impairments, use health services more frequently, are dissatisfied with the care offered, often suffer from alcohol abuse and complain of hypochondriasis. It is important that you consider what types of patients you find difficult to deal with, explore why you feel this way, and consider how you might learn to deal with them better.

Dying patients

When medical students and doctors have not come to terms with the idea that they could die at any time, or have not resolved their own previous bereavements, they may find it difficult to deal with the chronically ill and dying, give bad news and relate to the newly bereaved. There is a risk that they will become too detached or over-involved and then under- or over-treat the patient. Therefore you should ask the following questions.

- Has my own experience of loss and grief affected, enhanced or limited my ability to work with dying patients?
- What are my own attitudes towards death?
- How do my attitudes and concerns affect my ability to care for dying patients?
- If I were dying, what would I want and need from my doctor?

Medical mistakes

If medical students and doctors accept that medicine is a percentage business, aim to do their best, but recognize that they will not always be successful, and seek to learn from any mistakes, they will cope well. Those who believe they should be perfect and there is no room for mistakes will put undue pressure on themselves and consider themselves failures. This can result in a serious loss of self-esteem. They may become over-zealous about ordering tests and treatments to protect against the risk of failure. If they keep their worries hidden they will be especially at risk of burnout. Therefore, when mistakes occur it is important for you to consider the following questions.

- What is the nature of my mistake?
- What are my beliefs about my mistakes?
- What emotions do I experience?
- How did I cope?
- What changes did/or should I make in my practice?

DOCTORS' SELF-CARE

It is important that medical students and qualified doctors take steps to look after themselves and ensure their own emotional survival. Otherwise, constant exposure to stressors could seriously impair their effectiveness in relating to patients and colleagues. The questions for reflection mentioned above should lead to increased awareness and help you to maintain a more satisfying balance between your personal and professional lives. Medical students and doctors should constantly monitor their levels of stress, identify any key stresses and formulate ways in which they might deal with these. A particular challenge is to achieve a balance between one's personal and professional lives.

Doctors commonly complain that they have excessive workloads. While this may be beyond their control, it is often due to the fact that they are willing to take on too much. When they accept an excessive workload as inevitable, this can lead them to feel dissatisfied with their work, unhappy at home, and experience serious physical and emotional problems. When patients' demands increase and conflict develops at home, they may retreat still further into their work. Thus it is important to challenge assumptions such as 'work must come first', as it is possible for doctors to make choices about the balance in their lives and to avoid accepting the role of 'victim' or 'martyr'.

Medical students and doctors should set aside time to foster personal relationships, set clear goals for their lives, enjoy recreation and intellectual stimulation, and look for courses that will promote their professional development and confidence. They should ask themselves what their beliefs are about the ideal balance of time between work, play, family and personal development. They should consider whether there are major barriers to their achieving that balance, including the possibility that their own assumptions and behaviour are contributing to the problem. Are they aware of specific stresses in their lives? If so, can they find ways of coping with these more effectively?

A common problem is for doctors to deny that such stresses exist until they experience burnout or develop other serious problems. Therefore they should aim to set time aside for regular reflection and discussion to identify key stressors, strategies to manage those stressors, changes that they might need to make in their attitudes and behaviour, how they might better understand and improve their personal relationships, and how to arrange a better balance in relation to their priorities.

ENABLING PERSONAL SURVIVAL

Support and survival skills may be gained from one or more of the following:

- Peer support
- Discussion in small groups
- Balint groups
- Family-of-origin groups
- Personal awareness groups
- Developing communication skills

PEER SUPPORT

It may be sufficient for medical students and young doctors to talk to colleagues about these various questions in order to decide whether there are particular stressors that need attention, and to discuss the strategies they might use. This can be done effectively on an informal basis, although some medical schools now suggest peer counselling, where students are paired together to help each other cope with the stresses.

In the following example a student was experiencing undue distress when he encountered deaths on hospital wards. He asked a close medical student friend if he could talk to her about this. She explored how upset he was getting and confirmed that his distress seemed to be out of proportion. She asked him to reflect on whether he had gone through any previous losses himself that might explain why he was so distressed. He revealed that he had lost a beloved grandfather a few years ago. He had been unable to attend the funeral and felt very guilty about this, and he had suppressed his grief and never expressed it. As a result of this conversation with his fellow student he realized that he needed help and he sought counselling. The counselling enabled him to resolve his grief. He was then able to relate to dying patients and relatives much more effectively.

DISCUSSION IN SMALL GROUPS

Medical students ought to have opportunities to participate in small-group discussions about their clinical experiences and their associated concerns and feelings. The focus should be on the clinical care of patients, how patients have made them feel and the reasons for their reactions. They should also be asked if they have concerns about their relationships with other health professionals, and these concerns should be explored and discussed. The facilitator can then invite the medical students to consider the possible source of their feelings, so that they can make a connection between the feelings being provoked by their real-life experiences with patients and their own prior life experience. However, such groups should not become therapy groups. Instead, they should help students to realize how they can be affected by their patients, and that it is not 'pathetic' to experience distress. These groups can then consider what might be more useful strategies. Such groups can be supportive, but the matters discussed must be kept confidential within the group.

Such groups can also helpfully focus on any conflict that medical students and doctors are experiencing in relation to the care given to patients and relatives. For example, a student may be unhappy with the aggressiveness of a cancer therapy regime because he feels that the quality of life of the patient is being compromised without any likely benefits in terms of survival. It is not yet clear whether such groups should meet regularly or only when there has been some crisis in relation to patient care.

BALINT GROUPS

Some medical schools have introduced Balint-style groups for medical students and doctors. The aim is to ask participants to reflect on how they use 'themselves', as though they were the equivalent of a drug. How do they decide on the 'dose of themselves' that they give to patients and relatives? Are they giving too much or too little to particular types of patients, especially perhaps those whom they find challenging? What are the reasons behind this?

The aim of Balint groups is to help medical students and doctors to identify blind spots in their attitudes and behaviour – that is, issues related to them becoming over- or under-involved with patients of which they were not previously aware. The group can then help them to explore their attitudes and motivations in the hope that this will reduce their blind spots and make them more effective in their clinical practice.

FAMILY-OF-ORIGIN GROUPS

These are designed to help medical students and young doctors to obtain a better understanding of their strengths and blind spots by constructing personal genograms which depict the nature of the relationship with each member of the nuclear family. They are asked to highlight any conflicts, their roles in these relationships, the strengths and weaknesses of the family structure and the kinds of myths and expectations with which they grew up.

PERSONAL AWARENESS GROUPS

These are usually only offered to qualified doctors. They are unstructured, and a facilitator invites a group of 8 to 12 participants to reflect on any personal issues which they believe might have affected their ability to be effective as clinicians and teachers. For example, a senior female consultant reported that she had problems confronting a male colleague about his continued reluctance to break bad news and his tendency to give false reassurance. This was causing major conflict within the clinical team and leading to complaints from patients and relatives. Despite this, she could not bring herself to confront him.

When she discussed this problem in the group she became distressed. The facilitator invited her to consider where her fears of confronting him originated from. She disclosed that she was terrified that her male colleague would become aggressive towards her and try to destroy her. Her professional relationship with him would then be ruined. Members of the group were invited to reflect on whether or not they had similar fears of confrontation. Three other members of the group of eight did so. This legitimized the consultant's own fears and gave her the confidence to explore why she was so fearful.

She revealed that whenever she had tried to stand up to her father he had humiliated her. She was afraid that her colleague would also try to humiliate her, and she did not think she could deal with this. The group then suggested that, although her colleague was difficult, he might not react as badly as her father, particularly if she approached him in a constructive manner about the problems. She was able to do this and later reported a good outcome.

DEVELOPING COMMUNICATION SKILLS

Since difficulties in communicating with patients and relatives, particularly dying patients and bereaved relatives, are prominent among the reasons given for medicine being a stressful profession, it is crucial that medical students and doctors are equipped with the necessary communication skills, as discussed in previous chapters. Such training must include the opportunity to practise these key skills either in role play or with real patients or relatives, and to obtain constructive and enabling feedback from an experienced tutor who is knowledgeable about the skills and strategies that need to be learned.

Role play is particularly helpful in this context (Maguire *et al.*, 1996). A medical student or doctor is asked to play the part of a patient who has caused them concern in real life. For example, a student who had problems handling an angry patient may be invited to play that patient because the student will remember it vividly and should be able to portray the patient realistically. It will also give them an insight into the problem. Another medical student or doctor is then invited to play the interviewer who is trying to handle the anger.

The advantage of this approach is that the complexity of the task can be tailored to the level of experience of the student or doctor. Moreover, interviewers can be invited to stop as soon as they feel 'stuck', so that they are not humiliated in front of the group and made to feel deskilled. The group is then asked to suggest how the interview may be taken further and what strategies might work better.

The person playing the patient can then be invited to give feedback on how the different strategies suggested by the group worked in terms of whether it led to more disclosure, and how it made them feel generally. In this way, role play can become a series of experiments with the patient providing validation or refutation of the strategies that work best or fail to work. Medical students and doctors can then learn quickly and efficiently how to manage the situations with which they want help. When feedback is given, it is crucial that the group first comments on what the interviewer has done well, before any constructive criticisms are made. When those criticisms are subsequently made it is important that the person who is making the comment is also asked to give advice on what strategies might work better.

SUMMARY

If you are to learn to communicate effectively with your patients, you need to develop your self-awareness of what you find stressful, and the reasons for this. You will then be much better able to identify important stressors and find effective strategies to deal with them. This should reduce the risk of your developing burnout or even more severe psychological problems. Taking the trouble to improve your ability to handle areas of communication which you find difficult should do much to reduce the stress that you experience. It should also result in your receiving strong validation that patients like the way in which you communicate with them.

REFERENCES

Firth-Cousins, J. 1989: Stress in medical undergraduates and house officers. *British Journal of Hospital Medicine* **41**, 161–4.

Maguire, P., Booth, K., Elliott, C. and Jones, B. 1996: Helping health professionals involved in cancer care acquire key interviewing skills – the impact of the workshops. *European Journal of Cancer* **32A**, 1486–9.

Novack, D., Suchman, A.L., Clark, W., Epstein, R.M., Najberg, E. and Kaplan, C. 1998: Calibrating the physician: personal awareness and effective patient care. Working Group on Promoting Physician Personal Awareness. *Journal of the American Medical Association* **278**, 1657–8.

Ramirez, A., Graham, J., Richards, M.A. *et al.* 1995: Burnout and psychiatric disorder among cancer clinicians. *British Journal of Cancer* **71**, 1263–9.

INDEX

Page numbers in *italics* refer to figures.